ELECTRONIC
HEALTH
RECORDS

ELECTRONIC HEALTH RECORDS

STRATEGIES FOR LONG-TERM SUCCESS

MICHAEL FOSSEL | SUSAN DORFMAN

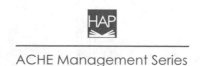

ACHE Management Series

Your board, staff, or clients may also benefit from this book's insight. For more information on quantity discounts, contact the Health Administration Press Marketing Manager at (312) 424–9470.

Library of Congress Cataloging-in-Publication Data
Fossel, Michael.
  Electronic health records : strategies for long-term success / by Michael Fossel and Susan Dorfman.
     pages cm
  ISBN 978-1-56793-560-8 (alk. paper)
1. Medical records–Data processing. I. Dorfman, Susan. II. Title.
  R864.F66 2013
  610.285–dc23
                         2012042012

The paper used in this publication meets the minimum requirements of American National Standard for Information Sciences—Permanence of Paper for Printed Library Materials, ANSI Z39.48-1984. ♾™

Acquisitions editor: Janet Davis; Project manager: Jennifer Seibert; Cover designer: Scott Miller; Layout: Fine Print, Ltd.

Found an error or a typo? We want to know! Please e-mail it to hapbooks@ache.org, and put "Book Error" in the subject line.

For photocopying and copyright information, please contact Copyright Clearance Center at www.copyright.com or at (978) 750–8400.

   Health Administration Press
   A division of the Foundation of the American
      College of Healthcare Executives
   One North Franklin Street, Suite 1700
   Chicago, IL 60606–3529
   (312) 424–2800

*To the physicians and nurses using EHRs daily,
who try to improve the lives of their patients
and deserve our support*

Contents

Foreword

I HAVE HAD the privilege of Michael Fossel's friendship for a number of years, and I can think of no better person to address the complexities of leading an information technology transition. His experience as a physician, researcher, and executive has given him a unique perspective on what is essentially an exercise in change management at, to use a biological term, the cellular level of an organization. As the complexity of healthcare delivery increases and public pressure mounts to reduce medical errors, Dr. Fossel and coauthor Susan Dorfman provide a road map for the conversion of our antiquated paper medical records to a modern electronic format that is incredibly timely and equally important.

The book addresses a number of key issues that are important to successfully converting to an electronic health record (EHR). The authors provide a comprehensive review that includes not only the basics of product selection and the logistics of project management but also the more subtle challenges of governance in the replacement of what is essentially the central nervous system of the modern hospital.

Because of their experience in medicine, information technology, and healthcare innovation, the authors also are able to speak to the challenges of changing ingrained behaviors. It is in this regard that they bring the most value to healthcare executives in the throes of an EHR conversion. In his book *Leadership Without Easy Answers*, Ronald Heifetz (1998) speaks to the challenges of change: "In human societies, adaptive work consists of efforts to close the gap between reality and a host of values not restricted to survival." In other words, conveying a need for change, communicating a vision for the future, and creating an infrastructure that will enable our teams to achieve that vision are some of our most important work as healthcare leaders. The EHR is the next generation of tools and technology that will allow our industry to move closer to the zero-defect environment that our patients and our communities should rightfully expect.

Doug Lawson, FACHE
Chief Operating Officer
Baylor University Medical Center
Dallas, Texas

Preface

THE ADVENT OF computers in medicine has been—for many providers—culturally jarring, politically difficult, and certainly expensive. While a number of factors have played a role in this current change, the original impetus was the understandable desire for better patient care. This desire evolved into the belief that we might not only improve patient care but also perhaps do so at a lower cost than has been the case. Over the past two decades, there has been a push to prevent avoidable medical errors and to lower the cost of care, and it has been strongly suggested that computers might help us accomplish these goals. Added to these goals is the need to meet the growing regulatory requirements of healthcare, especially since the advent of "meaningful use" criteria. The result is that almost all American—and most global— hospitals are transitioning from paper records to electronic health records (EHRs).

The Association of Medical Directors of Information Systems noted in its *Informatics Review* journal that the nationwide EHR implementation price tag is estimated at $150 billion over the coming eight years. Projections call for hospitals to spend $46 billion to acquire and expand their current EHR systems and another $55 billion in new operating costs. In every hospital, these costs have become a significant part of the annual budget. Projecting future costs and anticipating future regulatory hurdles are major goals of hospital leadership.

Our purpose is to make the transition easier and clearer. The experiences of the thousands of hospitals that have made this transition are universal; they share many of the same problems and develop many of the same solutions. Drawing from the stories of the hundreds of hospitals we have worked with, we describe how hospitals deal with new hardware and software; organize their governance; deal with their clinical staff; and manage their formularies, order sets, and documentation in the changing electronic world. The successes and failures, the right ways and wrong ways, the intuitive ways and the difficult ways of implementing a hospital EHR are not new; each hospital has—often by hit and miss—carved a unique path into the electronic world. This book offers insight into the pitfalls, problems, and peculiarities that occur along the way.

Our aim is not only to help you improve patient care—as well as help lower costs and meet regulatory goals—but also to ensure that you do so without the difficulties that others have had. Throughout, our advice is drawn from extensive experience; we hope that you can avoid some of our experiences and profit from the rest of them. Healthcare is in the midst of unparalleled change; we offer you a detailed view of that change and a map of how to survive it. Our strongest wish is to have all of us deliver not only different care, but better care.

PART I

Fundamentals

CHAPTER 1

Intent

The time has come for an electronic medical record in every
group medical practice in America. Period. End of story.

—*Donald Berwick*

WHY CONVERT?

No hospital should convert to an electronic health record (EHR)
simply to computerize care. Conversion is **not** a computer project;
it is a medical project that requires technical resources and technical support.

Computerizing a hospital is much like building a laboratory or
buying a new MRI machine: The goal is not to improve the hospital's pathology or radiology departments or its technology but
to improve the patient care it delivers. Technology is a tool, but it
isn't the goal. Too many hospitals view conversion as an information technology (IT) project with medical implications, which is
simply and disastrously **wrong**. It needs to be driven and governed
by a medical perspective, not an IT perspective.

Patient needs, compassionate care, better health, patient safety,
hospital finances, regulatory needs, ease of practice, medical costs,
and staff support are motivations that should underlie and drive
hospitals' decisions. Yet, hospitals sometimes put more money than
thought into their decisions. The purpose of hospitals—to provide
quality patient care—should underlie both the conversion and the
continuous optimization that occurs after the conversion.

There is more to providing quality patient care than meets the eye.

While many of us are unaware of it, the quality of medical care has been undergoing a revolution that is finally making itself felt and transforming medicine globally. A century ago, medical care in the United States and Canada was transformed by publication of the Flexner (1910) report *Medical Education in the United States and Canada*. Flexner condemned the quality of medical training in the United States and recommended that

- admission to medical school require applicants to have completed high school and two years of college focused on the study of basic science,
- medical students be required to complete four years of study in a curriculum approved by the Council on Medical Education, and
- medical schools be part of a university and have full-time clinical professors.

His report led to improved medical training that has become the envy of many other nations.

Yet over the past decade or so, the quality of care—especially in the United States, but globally as well—has been questioned and often found to be embarrassingly low. In 1999, the Institute of

Medicine released the infamous report *To Err Is Human: Building a Safer Health System*, decrying the prevalence of medical errors and recommending strategic changes in the organization and delivery of medical care at both the national level and in local hospitals and universities. The key point of those recommendations was not a better education but a better system:

> Preventing errors and improving safety . . . require a systems approach in order to modify the conditions that contribute to errors. People working in health care are among the most educated and dedicated workforce in any industry. The problem is not bad people; the problem is that the system needs to be made safer. (IOM 1999)

The problem is not that we lack knowledge, resources, intelligence, or training but rather that we lack the will and the understanding to transform the knowledge and resources into a system that can provide effective, compassionate care.

The key issue is not what we have but how we use it. Patients are injured not because we lack MRIs but because they wait needlessly, not because of a lack of surgical skill but because of a lack of organizational skill, and not from the dangers inherent in certain drugs but from our mistakes in prescribing and administering those drugs.

Most suggestions and prescriptions for improvement cite two themes: single-minded dedication to quality and more effective use of the tools we already have. Among these tools, the use of computers and information access are unanimously cited, not because computers **solve** our problems but because they **enable** us to solve our problems. It is not the computer itself that has value; rather, there is enormous value in our ability to access information, track and avoid errors, find what we need quickly and reliably, make decisions, and implement care without error or delay. At their worst, computers can, as one pharmacist said, "let us make mistakes faster than ever"; at their best, computers can help us achieve a level of quality care we could never achieve without them. But they cannot help us if we do not have a single, clear goal: **quality. No mistakes, no delays, and no exceptions.**

Computers are not the end, yet they can be the **means** to achieving our end: a total transformation of patient care. How can we effectively transform both our hospitals and ourselves? Part of that transformation—and if done well, the most effective part—is moving our hospitals into a world of informed decisions, errorless

---

Did You Know?

Only one in seven medical errors is recognized and reported in US hospitals. The Inspector General estimates that more than 130,000 Medicare patients experience one or more adverse events in hospitals per month (Sweeney 2012).

---

therapy, and seamlessly integrated medical care: a world that makes optimal use of computers.

Bringing a hospital into the computer age is easy; doing so successfully is much harder. The difficulty lies not in the technical complexity—turning software into a clinical tool—but in the human complexity: converting **people**. We must ask people to change the way they do what they do and then continually modify, tweak, and optimize it. To reprogram computers is straightforward; to reprogram human beings is a daunting but necessary challenge. People need to learn and relearn, evaluate and reevaluate, make decisions and remake even better decisions.

Converting hospitals requires careful planning; converting people requires patience, hard work, a good understanding of human nature, and a sense of humor. To practice medicine, we need a compassionate understanding of reality; the same is true when converting people. To be a good social worker, a good psychologist, or a good politician, we must have our feet on the ground while keeping our eyes on the sky. Successful conversion requires no less. We need to understand the nitty-gritty of the hardware, the complexities of the software, and the realities of medical care; equally, we need to understand **why** we are converting in the first place. The rationale for conversion and subsequent changes may seem obvious, but too often it is not. Statements of purpose—the vision, the goal, and the point of the process—commonly are no more than wishful thinking, and sometimes bad thinking at that.

> **Tip**
>
> Training is crucial to converting hospitals and people and to ensuring utilization. It is also tied to federal incentive payments requiring that healthcare providers and workers meaningfully use the system. Some doctors, nurses, and healthcare workers doubt the benefits of EHRs, particularly for improving the care of their patients and even their own productivity. A broad range of approaches can be taken to get them on board and fully participating, including a combination of peer-to-peer training sessions, online and offline sessions to meet custom schedules and needs, assignment of executive sponsors and team leads, and even components of competitive gaming, such as team or individual leader boards.

DEFINING A VISION

In many organizations, the vision statement is window dressing. It is made to please the public relations department and crafted to ease the politically correct. It is calligraphy for the organization's website and nothing more. The hypocrisy is exposed in the veiled sarcasm of physician staff and the eye-rolling of staff nurses when no administrators are present: "*Sure* they believe in better patient care, as long as it doesn't involve helping *my* patients." While these colleagues do need a vision—an honest one—they also have a vision of their own that keeps them coming to work, one that drives the professionals in any well-run hospital.

A vision statement should **be** concrete, and it also should inspire concrete **results**. Although it is only an informal motto, the Royal Canadian Mounted Police's famous claim "We always get our man" must have given pause to many a potential lawbreaker and made it easier for the force to meet its formal motto *Maintiens* *le droit* ("maintain the law"). The US Postal Service, its function now increasingly undercut by e-mail and the erosion of established communication patterns, once was driven by the unofficial motto "Neither snow nor rain nor heat nor gloom of night stays these couriers from the swift completion of their appointed rounds." The fact that this "vision statement" was unofficial and plagiarized from Herodotus's description of the Persian courier service did not undermine the respect it engendered for the postal service of a young nation. In the popular culture of times past, the postman, especially the rural postman, was an example to emulate.

In the case of hospitals, **an accurate, credible vision can have measurable effects on EHR implementation and optimization, reimbursement, and patient survival rates.**

Example of Success: Hospital #1

One example of success comes from a large medical center in the Midwest that achieved total compliance with computerized physician order entry (CPOE), largely because of the center's vision and the way in which it was applied.

Tip

For a hospital to realize its vision, members of the hospital staff must be able to answer three key questions:

1. How do you see yourself practicing medicine within the next five years?
2. What objectives and goals does the hospital vision incorporate to enable you to do so?
3. What tools and systems can help you and your peers achieve those goals and objectives?

Keep in mind that success depends on each person's ability to tie the vision to concrete, personal actions.

In converting its eight hospitals—a combination of community and academic, inner city and suburban, general and specialty—the center kept to a single, firm vision: **improving patient care**. This goal was consistently hammered into staff at all levels; the management team meant it and made it stick. The mantra of improving patient care was not empty fluff, a mere "framed message," or saccharine hypocrisy; it was concrete and inarguable. The message underlying the vision could be summed up in three concepts:

1. We can use computers and CPOE to improve our patient care.
2. If you don't agree, tell us why so we can make it work.
3. If you still don't want to use the system, you must not value patient care—in which case, why are you practicing here?

Many physicians and nurses faced with EHR issues (and, historically, any other hospital issue) use the trump card of patient care: They claim that a given change will compromise patient care. Because quality of care is ultimately a medical evaluation rather than an administrative one, their claim is difficult to challenge, absent good objective data. In this case, the center preempted the trump card and communicated a clear message: *If we all are trying to improve patient care, you should be helping improve, rather than obstructing, our project.* Staff couldn't easily evade this statement: Go along with the project and help fix problems, or leave. The center achieved 100 percent compliance, both initially and over the ensuing years as it strove to optimize patient care.

Defining Goals to Support the Vision

A supported, consistent vision is overwhelming and inescapable and drives a hospital to achieve what it could never achieve otherwise. Beyond a vision—even a concrete, credible one—we must define reasonable, achievable, and measurable goals that support that vision.

A clear understanding of our goals enables us to plot our course, correct our mistakes, and measure our success—if we have succeeded at all. We may have a vision, but the purpose of clearly stating our goals is to understand **why** we are doing what we do, **how** to achieve our goals, and **whether** we have succeeded when we finish. If we can't see and measure concrete benefits, our vision is mere words. It is sterile.

The goal isn't to convert to an electronic world or to install a pretty interface. It is deeper and more difficult to attain. What is the point of installing that interface? Until we understand our goal, we risk spending money and using resources only to achieve something that no one wanted in the first place.

When we convert a hospital, what is our goal? Why bother?

Is our goal better patient care, patient safety, improved financial return, staff satisfaction, or regulatory compliance? IT is an **enabler**; at best, it can help you **reach** your goal, but it should not **be** your goal. Likewise, when we evaluate a system, we should not focus on its features but on the **usability** of those features. Do they improve patient care? Do they make us safer? Faster? Better?

A computer may **enable** us to document in exquisite detail, but do staff actually **use** it to document effectively and efficiently? A computer may record every order and warn us about medical errors, but can staff place those orders in the midst of providing compassionate patient care? Will those warnings improve patient care, or will staff ignore the warnings because they are too frequent, too intrusive, or mindlessly confusing? A computer may offer us generous displays of patient information, but in that glut of data, will we be able to find the details we need in time to make the best clinical decision?

The key question is not "What is a **system** capable of?" but rather "What will a system make **us** capable of?"

Once we know our goals, a good system must support those goals. It must protect our patients and staff, promote good care and caring, lower our costs and our patients' costs, and enable us to improve what we do; otherwise, it is not worth installing. Some hospitals forget this crucial point—or act as though they have. They concentrate on features, aesthetics, or a narrow regulatory interest to the neglect of their mission, staff, and patients. Neither aesthetics nor a narrow attention to legal pressures is a sufficient reason for converting, and neither contributes to the project's credibility—an element essential to recruiting clinical staff to support such systems or, indeed, such hospitals. If physicians, nurses, and other clinical staff perceive the rationale for conversion as purely a reaction to legislation or finance—and even more important, if it is perceived as a purely executive decision made behind closed doors and without consultation—they will not support the system.

Getting physicians and nurses to use a system is often compared (like so much of human behavior) to "herding cats," and the only effective way to herd cats—or clinical staff—is to convince the majority of them to move in the direction we have in mind. The best (and only reliable) way to do so is to use their own motivations. In the hospital environment, the most common motivation shared

---

Motivation and Drive

I once asked a medical student about his motivation to become a doctor. Without doing much thinking, he honestly replied that his motivation was professional and financial security and then continued by expressing his drive to enhance patients' lives. That's when it hit me: the difference between motivation and drive. I thought about the many doctors, nurses, and other medical staff who practice in countries such as Russia, India, and China and even in some underserved regions in the United States, where dedication to patient care outweighs any financial benefit, and it became increasingly clear to me that healthcare professionals are ultimately driven to their field not primarily out of financial motivation but more so by their determination to help others.

—Susan Dorfman

---

by staff is to provide good patient care. Although many of us forget our altruistic goals in our day-to-day battles with the insertion of central lines, scheduling, The Joint Commission, and litigation risk, the urge to provide good care remains active. We follow this urge back to the hospital for our next shift instead of looking for a job elsewhere.

Patient care is why we work in a hospital and not in an accounting office. At some level, most of us—excited by our quotidian jobs or not, happy to admit it or not—care about the patients we serve. We work hard to provide compassionate, quality care to those patients. And our vocations and colleagues matter to us. These bonds hold a hospital together and inspire staff to convert from the world of paper to the world of computers and then continually improve it thereafter.

We have already considered the case of a large medical center whose vision—improving patient care—enabled its continuing success. Consider what happens when the opposite occurs. A hospital can make one of three mistakes in this regard:

1. It lacks a defined vision.
2. It has a vision that no one believes.
3. It never carries through on its vision.

The first error is the least common of the three; most hospitals make some attempt to define their *raison d'être*, even if it remains in brochures or in the tiny print on an obscure web page.

The second error occurs when the vision is well defined and even well publicized but the staff regards the vision as a window dressing. Effective visions are not the creation of a public relations consultant.

The third error occurs when the vision is credible but nothing happens. A good vision can (and probably should) be slightly ahead of reality, but it cannot be independent of reality. A slight disparity (we're good, but we want to be even better) is effective as long as hospitals carry through and catch up. The hospital must not only state the vision; it must intend to achieve it.

Example of Failure: Hospital #2

A nationwide hospital system (of almost three dozen facilities) converted to an EHR but neglected to link its vision (the essence of which was to "create excellent patient care," although the actual statement was turgid) to the changing use of computers in its hospitals. Physicians did not have a clear (let alone consistent) idea of the rationale for conversion, so they invented several. A majority of them attributed the change to the system CEO's friendship with his golf partner, whose cousin was the CEO of the EHR vendor. This belief was the explanation they gave for both the project itself and the choice of vendor.

The fact that this rationale was a fabrication is not the point; the physicians weren't consulted about the project, so they felt it was not done to "create excellent patient care" and was therefore not worth supporting. The vision was apt, but it didn't connect with the reality of the hospital wards and the medical staff. They also felt it did not reflect the reality of management's behavior.

The outcome was not only poor support but wholesale obstruction by many of the medical staff. Even those who supported the use of computers and cutting-edge IT complained about the project and resented that the system was forcing them to use computers. Compliance was low and backslides occurred frequently—a marked contrast to the outcomes achieved by the medical center described earlier in the chapter.

Lacking a vision, having a discredited vision, and not linking the vision to reality are all causes of failure. In the absence of information, people create folklore; in the absence of a vision, people create rumors.

A vision is not words on a web page. A vision commands truth, intent, and follow-through. A credible vision is important to the day-to-day success of a hospital and even more so when we fundamentally change the way we do that day-to-day work. To implement and optimize an electronic approach to medical care, we must have a map. The map must be accurate, and we must follow it. Our vision is that map.

DEFINING BENEFITS

Implementation is one thing, but defining success and optimizing usage are quite another. We not only need a map—our vision; we also need to be able to measure how far we are from our path and whether we are moving in the right direction. To do so we must define the benefits we wish to attain, and those benefits must be congruent with our overarching vision. It is all very well to have a vision of "good patient care" (who doesn't?), but what exactly is good patient care? Is it related to the rate of readmission, the rate of complications, Press Ganey scores, length of stay, bed occupancy, regulatory compliance, or financial numbers? Is it all of these measures (and dozens of others) or some weighted calculation derived from them? A number of factors that contribute to good patient care are difficult to measure; should they be included in our definition?

Defining benefits yields several benefits of its own.

We can align our departments and staffs, enabling us to settle squabbles and increase efficiency when comparing "apples to oranges." Should we install several new servers or buy a new MRI instead? How do we resolve the conflicting trade-offs between efficient radiology department billing and the efficient workflow of the clinical physicians who are trying to order the radiology studies? For example, while radiology may find it expedient to use a name that is convenient for billing purposes (e.g., "NV" for a Doppler study), the clinical physicians who order the study find this nomenclature obscure and confusing. Would we rather have scribes or an effective word recognition dictation system? Trade-offs are endless but easier to untangle if we know what we are trying to accomplish.

If end users understand the benefits of the new technology in tangible, concrete terms relevant to their daily work, they are more likely to support the change. It is easier to understand how the role of a ward secretary or a triage nurse will change—and how to train that individual for that modified role—once we clearly understand what we are trying to accomplish. Defining our benefits helps us define how we use our clinical personnel effectively. It is not enough to merely have a rationale; the defined benefits must be continually applicable and obtainable at all levels of your organization.

Defining benefits is not a naïve process. They are useful only if they

1. are measurable,
2. are the right measures,
3. are measures that can be changed, and
4. are supported by both pre- and post-conversion data or continual data.

The first characteristic seems obvious, yet most of us have had the experience of sitting through committee meetings defining enviable but nebulous benefits such as "better patient care," "greater compassion," and "better efficiency." While all of these benefits are desirable, they are not defined—and may not be definable in many cases. A benefit need not be expressed in mathematically sophisticated terms, but it does need to be quantified. If 90 percent of our patients agree that our care is "much better" than before project implementation, we may not know precisely what our patients mean, but this outcome is still desirable. If we can't measure benefits, however informally, we can't tell if we are improving.

The second characteristic also seems obvious, yet we see the opposite every day. The problem is that we tend to choose easily measured "markers" as substitutes for the true benefits, which are less easily measured. For example, we hate to have patients waiting unnecessarily in the emergency department (ED), so we choose to measure length of stay (LOS) because we want to minimize it. In general, this marker is adequate, but it would be naïve to interpret it without looking at other measures. In the absurd extreme, we could easily reduce LOS to zero simply by discharging all patients prior to evaluation or treatment—a perfect LOS, but the worst possible patient care. In short, LOS is a useful marker, but it needs to be balanced against other, equally useful markers, such as regulatory compliance, adequacy of evaluation, and medical outcome. LOS is only a stand-in marker—and certainly not the only such marker—for the more important, overarching benefits that are

---

Using the Wrong Marker

In the 1990s, a cardiac drug was touted for significantly lowering serum cholesterol. Serum cholesterol was a widely used clinical measure of drug efficacy, but in this case, it was the wrong one. The drug may have lowered patients' cholesterol, but it also markedly increased their mortality. After numerous deaths were linked to the drug, it was taken off the market, despite the earlier encomiums.

remarkably hard to measure directly, such as "quality of care." Any benefit measure must be interpreted in a broader clinical context, and few, if any, can be held as single, independent measures of our greater goals.

Third, we need to be able to change what we measure. Some measurements might improve if we didn't have to meet regulatory guidelines, but we do. Others might improve if we stopped delivering a service line, increased our investment in capital items, or hired more full-time equivalents (FTEs), but these changes are not always feasible or appropriate. Measure what you can change, not what you can't change. Benefits measurement should open an opportunity, not increase our frustration.

Fourth, useful measures comprise data from more than one point in time; they illustrate a trend. If, after converting to CPOE, we find that we have a 1 percent rate of medication error, does this information indicate a growing disaster or a vast improvement over our previous (unknown) rate of error? It is often difficult to obtain data on events prior to a conversion because we may need to have an electronic system to gather certain data in the first place. Equally, we may have data that don't imply anything useful, such as the compliance rate with CPOE prior to instituting CPOE. Before CPOE, compliance was obviously zero. In either case, comparison of pre- and post-conversion measures does not yield useful information, but comparing data over time does. We can track physician compliance with CPOE over the first several weeks after implementation and look for a trend. If, for example, we have no record of the number of times the wrong antibiotic was ordered pre-CPOE because no one wrote it down and a paper audit would be too costly, we can gather data over time after conversion. A strong downward trend in inappropriate antibiotic choice during the first 12 months is a benefit, regardless of the number of incorrect antibiotic prescriptions written prior to the conversion.

Having viewed potential benefit measures "from 35,000 feet," let's finish at ground level with examples of specific benefits.

The goal is **not** to measure every possible benefit but to focus on a cluster of key benefits. Typically, a hospital CPOE implementation focuses on a dozen (or fewer) benefits, while an ED implementation focuses on half a dozen (or fewer) benefits. The following list includes examples of benefit measures for an ED implementation:

- ED throughput—meaningful use
- Resource time to track 72-hour returns to ED
- Accounts receivable days
- ED reimbursement and total charge capture
- Capture of wait times (e.g., door to doctor)
- LOS for patients discharged from ED

Here is an extensive list of potential hospital-wide benefit measures:

- Clinical measures
  - —Operating room turnaround time (TAT)
  - —LOS (inpatient and ED separately)
  - —Monthly LOS per Diagnosis-Related Group (DRG) of interest
  - —TAT from lab order to result documentation (both stat/now and routine types)
  - —Number of adverse drug events per 100 admissions
  - —TAT from medication order to administration
  - —Intensive care unit (ICU) LOS
  - —ED LOS
  - —TAT from blood order to first administration
  - —Number of ventilator days per ICU stay
  - —Mortality rate per DRG
  - —Complication rate per DRG
  - —ICU mortality rate
  - —Infection rate (e.g., per year, per unit)
  - —Missed or delayed orders (e.g., medications, EKG)

- System measures
  - Percentage of physicians using CPOE
  - Downtimes (e.g., frequency, duration)
  - Number of order sets used per admission or per physician
  - Percentage of radiology orders with completed "reason for exam"
  - Percentage of consult orders with completed "reason for consult"
  - Number of RN calls requesting clarification of orders
  - Time required for physician to write orders (e.g., post-op)
  - Percentage of orders placed using CPOE
  - Percentage of orders placed by each communication type
  - Clicks per order
  - System speed
    - Response time per click
    - Time to view labs
    - Time to view diagnostic studies
    - Time to view documents
- Financial measures
  - Increased revenue per financial quarter
  - Revenue: charges per ED visit
  - Gross visit-level charges: use of proper coding
  - Total cost per discharge for DRGs of interest
  - Use of automated protocols/guidelines to reduce expensive variations in medications (therapeutic substitutions)
- Regulatory compliance measures
  - ED compliance with ED core measures
  - Fall risk assessment
  - Pressure ulcers present on admission
  - Delinquent charges
  - Delayed order signing
  - Pain assessments after medication
  - Joint Commission core measures for acute myocardial infarction, community-acquired pneumonia, congestive heart failure, and pregnancy

KEY POINTS

- Conversion is **not** a computer project; it is a medical project.
- **Define a vision**:
  —Make it reflect the reality of your reasons for converting.
  —Communicate it at all levels.
  —Maintain and enforce it.
- **Define benefits** that are (1) measurable, (2) accurate measures of your goal, and (3) attainable, and measure them over time.

CHAPTER 2

Vendors, Consultants, and Changing Systems

*What is a cynic? A man who knows the price
of everything and the value of nothing.*

—*Oscar Wilde*

EVALUATING A SYSTEM

The key issue is not price, but value.

The exception, of course, is if you can't afford the price. Hence, capital budget permitting, the primary question to consider when choosing an EHR is: Does it provide the best value for the money?

Hospital budgets are complicated; difficult and unpredictable trade-offs must be made. If we add three med/surg nurses at roughly a quarter of a million dollars per year, we may reduce the number of patients who return after discharge but we will either increase or decrease the hospital's profit, depending on the current regulatory climate, baseline patient returns, and the split between nonpayers, Medicare/Medicaid patients, and private-pay patients.

EHRs are at least as complicated as anything else in the hospital world. When hiring nurses, we can—with some accuracy— predict what those nurses are capable of doing. Electronic systems are less predictable. They are still relatively new and rapidly changing (hopefully improving), so it is often hard to tell which ones do what functions and which would provide the most value in our particular hospital, vendor claims notwithstanding. Often we find ourselves looking backward after installation and wishing we had known beforehand what we came to know afterward. EHRs are not, however, as unpredictable as the regulatory climate, which usually changes with each presidential election and becomes even stricter—and certainly more costly—than the current climate.

Electronic health systems may change as much as regulations do, but they improve—if slowly and fitfully—which is more than can be unequivocally said of regulatory burdens. Over time, they are becoming more functional and more useful. Moreover, certain observations are clear about these systems:

- Hospital-wide systems are gradually replacing niche systems.
- All major systems can access data, place orders, and support documentation.
- Most systems now offer decision support, reports, and additional features.
- Systems' ease of use varies; some are more intuitive than others.
- Vendors vary in experience and in support capabilities.

OUR GOALS

Before exploring these observations—and the vendors—we need to hold fast to our goals. We cannot evaluate a vendor or select

---

Placing a Value on EHRs

"Health IT is the foundation for a truly 21st century health system where we pay for the right care, not just more care," said US Department of Health & Human Services' Secretary Kathleen Sebelius in a February 2012 news release. Physicians, nurses, and hospitals should be taking advantage of this unique opportunity to implement new, smarter systems that improve patient care and create "the jobs we need for an economy built to last."

---

a system if we lose sight of our intent: Why are we installing an EHR? EHRs are more than electronic, more than health, and more than records. They substantially change processes, affect all aspects of care, and enable us not only to record information but also to access data, place orders, (potentially) improve safety, and use current knowledge to improve decision making.

If we buy EHRs to improve patient care or to meet regulatory requirements, they need to meet these goals. We cannot purchase just any system or a flashy interface. Before assessing an EHR, we need to state—seriously and in some detail—the grounds for making our assessment: What do we expect the system and the vendor to do for us? Can the system do what we want? Can the vendor install and support the system we want?

NICHE SYSTEMS: "THE BEST OF BREED"

In the early 2000s, the market offered a large number of "niche" systems. Typically, these systems grew out of the needs of a single department or specialty and—because they were designed by and for the physicians in that department/specialty—generally did a fine job of meeting their particular needs.

Compare Needs, Not Features

The first error hospitals make when evaluating EHR systems is to use a checklist approach to compare **vendors.**

→ **Wrong:** comparing vendors according to the features they offer

→ **Right:** comparing your needs to the features vendors offer

Don't compare **vendors;** compare your **needs** to the solutions vendors offer.

The market for niche systems, once healthy, is gradually being eroded by vendors who offer comprehensive, hospital-wide systems. The reasons for this shift in the market are complex, but three factors predominate: (1) Niche systems don't always "play well" with other systems in other hospital departments, (2) hospitals (rather than departments) are now making most of the purchasing decisions, and (3) regulatory requirements are increasingly affecting entire hospitals rather than individual departments. Niche vendors (no matter how well they may have met the needs of that niche until now) are gradually disappearing, and the market is moving toward whole-hospital systems supplied by only a handful of large national—and international—vendors.

For the emergency department setting, for example, scores of niche systems have been developed, of which only a handful have competed in the national market. These niche systems were designed by emergency physicians and generally have been responsive to the needs of that market. They are adaptable to change, have intuitive interfaces, and are well loved by their users. Although they rarely meet the larger needs of hospitals, emergency physicians strongly prefer them because they are easy to use and support the physician workflow in the emergency department.

Similar niche systems serving parallel needs cropped up in other specialties, including surgery, labor and delivery, general ambulatory care, family practice, and ophthalmology. With few exceptions, all successful niche systems have shared two general characteristics: (1) They were designed by practitioners in the specialty for which they were developed, and (2) they have met the workflow needs of those specialty practitioners.

Niche Systems Lose Market Share

Niche systems—often successful, well designed, and laudable—have a common drawback that has limited their market: They don't interface well with the rest of the hospital and cannot be easily cobbled together with other such systems to build a unified hospital system. The "best of breed" approach has often resulted in a "worst of breed" outcome.

Emergency niche systems, for example, may not easily access laboratory results or radiology images. Those that can access such data may not be able to place medication orders. Some can place orders but can't bill for those medications. Some retain records within the emergency department but can't be readily accessed by other departments. Many can't handle nursing functions at all.

Despite such limitations, niche systems have maintained a loyal following among many specialists because they make their lives—and their clinical work—much easier. Some of these systems are remarkably sophisticated and their functionality hard to outperform. They may be superb at meeting regulatory guidelines, obtaining consults, generating reports, or minimizing wasted time or patient risk—but only in a single department.

Instead of growing larger to encompass other specialties and add hospital-wide functions, niche players have remained localized to a single specialty and are quickly losing market to hospital-wide systems. Moreover, most hospital-wide system vendors have shown little interest in buying the niche players or in adapting the features of these remarkably adept systems to their products.

LARGE-VENDOR SYSTEMS

As discussed earlier, most of the market for hospital-wide systems is held by a handful of large vendors (e.g., Cerner, Epic). These vendors began by developing niche systems and have grown and taken over the market by broadening their systems' abilities. Cerner's EHR began as a laboratory system and grew to accommodate the needs of entire hospitals, including ambulatory venues; Epic's EHR began as an ambulatory system and also grew to take on the needs of whole hospitals, including inpatient venues. In 2010, there were 210 known EHR vendors. Depending on our definitions, we might realistically claim that the North American market is controlled by three major vendors and eight other significant vendors. Many vendors are now global, and a few are found only outside North America.

Because purchasing decisions are now generally made—and because regulatory requirements are generally applied—at the institutional level rather than at the departmental level, these major vendors design systems that meet the needs of the entire hospital and are not driven by physician needs per se, let alone the needs of any single department. Major vendors purport to offer a single, integrated, seamless, hospital-wide system that supports multiple functions, including access to clinical data, management of orders, and clinical documentation (and often other capacities).

Despite the shift toward hospital-wide systems, the needs of clinical personnel—whether driving the market or not—must be kept in focus for two reasons:

1. The core mission of the hospital is not regulatory or fiscal but clinical, and physicians and nurses represent (or most closely represent) this mission.
2. Successful implementation requires adoption by all clinical personnel, including physicians, nurses, and other staff.

Hospital-wide systems must account for these basic needs within the context of the hospital's overall, usually broader needs (e.g., fiscal, regulatory, political) and vision.

THE CLINICAL PERSPECTIVE

While the primary clinical requirements of an EHR are workflow support and an intuitive, efficient interface, the way in which physicians and nurses view (and use) the interface needs to be understood. Clinical personnel often break down the basic functions of EHR systems into three categories: viewing data, placing orders, and documenting care (sometimes seen as sensory, motor, and memory functions). Other clinical requirements include decision support (e.g., which antibiotic would be most appropriate for a particular patient), regulatory reminders or enforcement (e.g., whether aspirin was given on admission of a patient with a myocardial infarction), prevention of medical errors (e.g., warning the physician of a drug allergy), and dynamic differential diagnosis or appropriate order suggestions. Almost all major vendors offer a combined suite that handles the basic three clinical functions, but the inclusion of additional support functions varies among them.

A purely clinical perspective does not consider other functions that are critical to the hospital, including billing, registration, scheduling, inventory, and reporting. To varying degrees of success, most vendors meet these needs as well. Evaluation of any vendor system must consider its ability to support the entire spectrum of patient care within the venue of the institution. Evaluation based on ability to support a single clinical department (e.g., labor and delivery) or a single function (e.g., billing) is insufficient. Moreover, it is becoming increasingly important that a system communicate with other systems, both within and between hospitals. While many hospitals are struggling to meet state laws requiring them to interface—or at least share data—with immunization registries, others are simply trying to participate in national clinical registries (such as the trauma registry). Data sharing—with appropriate restrictions—is only going to increase as hospitals expect to trade information with other hospitals and as patients store their personal medical data in commercial databases (such as those of Microsoft). Local, regional, state, and even global databases are under discussion (and not always supportively); in the future, hospitals will expect their software to meet data interface needs that are yet to be defined.

Even when two vendors offer roughly equivalent functions, important differences determine success and the hospital's return on investment. A system that offers every possible function may have a clumsy interface and be difficult to learn, resulting in grudging or minimal compliance among the hospital staff. The best of systems is useless when your staff refuses to use it. System selection

Food for Thought

The perceived ease of use of any system is the result of three factors:

1. The hospital's medical and political leadership
2. Clinical staff's age or computer experience
3. Characteristics of the interface

Specific issues to consider when assessing clinical ease of use include

- the number of keystrokes required per order (e.g., EKG, antibiotic),
- the use of synonyms/generics (e.g., for labs, radiology, drugs),
- the depart process (How intuitive, supportive, and efficient is it?),
- drug reconciliation (rapid, high percentage of matches),
- order sets (easy to modify and reflect actual clinical workflow),
- departmental or individual favorites (to enable rapid ordering),
- nursing documentation (ease of entry and later readability),
- nursing tasks (driving workflow without being onerous),
- regulatory support (for current and upcoming requirements),
- linked or complex orders (e.g., blood bank, total parenteral nutrition, oncology), and
- reporting (for quality assurance, clinician efficacy, and risk behaviors).

based on published rankings of physicians' vendor preferences does not guarantee acceptance, either. Physicians may respond to fashion, hearsay, and system appearance as well as to long-term usability. Some systems get low ratings from staff initially or when only portions have been installed but are highly rated once the entire suite is in place and physicians gain experience with it. Curiously, a system may be intensely disliked in one hospital and highly valued in another, otherwise identical hospital.

Put bluntly, a poor interface will do well in a hospital with the "right" attitude, while a superb interface will fail in a hospital with an angry medical staff. The political and social issues that create success are discussed in later chapters, but two points must be made at this juncture: (1) Success is not simply a matter of a good interface, but (2) vendors' products differ markedly in their ease of use. User-friendliness is often subjective and hard to assess, and in the face of competition, vendors actively change and refine their interfaces. Systems' intuitiveness has improved noticeably over the past several years, and this refinement can be expected to continue. All of the above caveats notwithstanding, a user-friendly interface will increase your chances of converting successfully.

Laws of Good Electronic Health Records

- A perfect system wouldn't require staff training; poor designs require more training.
- Good care results from good clinical training, not from good IT training.
- Anything you type twice is typed one time too many.
- Two clicks are too many clicks.
- A good system supports the way we **actually** think and the way we **really** practice.
- A good EHR promotes—rather than interferes with— good patient care.

EVALUATING VENDORS

Functionality and ease of use are not the only important differences between systems. Factors independent of the system are also critical to consider:

- Which vendor has more experience with installation?
- Which vendor will offer better support after installation?

None of us wants to be the first to adopt a system—however highly touted—from a vendor who has never done an installation, nor do we want to install a system and then have the vendor walk away the next day. These issues—experience and support—are now magnified: With an estimated $35 billion in financial incentives at stake, hospitals are under enormous pressure to meet regulatory requirements and meaningful-use criteria and to install EHRs that will quickly and effectively enable them to do so.

Can vendors meet the demand? Even if a vendor has done a thousand installations and has a good reputation for providing technical support, can it realistically take on the enormous number of clients suddenly demanding new systems? Do they have the technical depth and the number of employees necessary to meet the needs of the market?

Impact in Numbers

A 2012 report by The Advisory Board Company and HIMSS Analytics shows a growing percentage of US hospitals at each Electronic Medical Record Adoption Model (EMRAM) stage. In 2008, twenty-eight hospitals achieved Stage 6 status, and fourteen achieved Stage 7. By the fourth quarter of 2011, two hundred seventy-seven hospitals had achieved Stage 6 status and sixty-five had achieved Stage 7.

CHOOSING A VENDOR PARTNER

Vendors differ, but our criteria for evaluation should remain consistent. A good vendor is a partner that shares an honest interest in our mutual success. Most hospitals share project goals—and are partners—with their vendors. This cultural characteristic not only greatly increases the odds of implementing a system successfully but also fosters a better professional work environment. However, some hospitals have a competitive, or even a malicious, view of their vendor, which markedly decreases their likelihood of achieving success. In most cases, the problem resides with the hospital's culture and is present long before a vendor is considered; in other cases, the problem begins the moment the vendor arrives and may be part of the vendor's culture.

While hospitals and vendors vary widely across this spectrum, and while it may be impossible to alter a hospital's prevailing culture, the hospital can choose a vendor that has a cooperative culture—one that will partner, not patronize.

Third-Party Consultants

A similar mistake sometimes occurs when a third party is brought on board. While many third parties contribute to a project's success, it often depends on why the third party is hired and how the third party interacts with the hospital and the vendor.

In the worst case, the third party is brought on board to "crack the whip" or "keep the vendor in line." This attitude reveals the malice and distrust inherent in the hospital and **cannot be changed** by a third-party consultant. In my experience, these same hospitals deride the "union mentality" of their staffs, and tellingly, these hospitals have a long, profitless history of disputes. They bring the same mind-set to new vendor relationships, and they intend to "win" by using the third party as a bludgeon. A "hired gun" merely compounds the problem, however: If you need a consultant to keep your vendor in line, who will keep your consultant in line? Third parties never should be brought in to serve as police; if a hospital's existing culture is unhealthy, compounded of paranoia and anger, a third party will never solve the inherent problems. Nothing will. There is no substitute for a healthy culture and a vendor that is part of the team.

In the best case, a third-party consultant—and there are many good ones—is brought in to complement the vendor's abilities by providing what the vendor cannot. If the vendor is weak at training, project management, managing order sets, or performing other critical parts of the transition to the EHR, the third party may supply a high return on investment. Sometimes the third party may be more of a technical advisor than a project manager; IBM, for example, has occasionally served in this role. Hire third-party consultants only when they can provide services that your vendor cannot provide or cannot provide as efficiently, as well, or as cheaply.

Some vendors offer "full service" in an attempt to become value-added business partners rather than merely technical advisors and software suppliers. Recognizing that the US implementation market will reach saturation point in the next several years, vendors are transitioning from software to consultant organizations and offering other services—such as remote hosting, data mining, clinical decision support, and revenue and collection services—to gain a competitive edge. For example, one major vendor has ten times more clinical consultants than any other vendor has.

The key point is: Do **not** hire a third party to control your vendor. If you can't be partners with your vendor, you probably can't be partners with your consultant either.

Evaluation Criteria

When we are evaluating a vendor, our primary consideration is the vendor's ability to provide the services we require and to maintain a good working relationship. Does the vendor

1. offer the features we need (as opposed to just offering more features)?

2. have an installation base—in users or hospitals—that makes it credible?
3. provide software known to be reliable?
4. offer the services we need to get the software up and running?
5. offer to support us after conversion, with both upgrades and issues?
6. offer a system known to be user-friendly for physicians, nurses, and other staff?
7. have other clients who can affirm its claims?
8. have a history that suggests it will still be around in a decade?
9. provide a good return on investment, given its cost?

The first question is often the most difficult because many hospitals struggle to define exactly what they want from an EHR. Overall, an EHR is an approach to better medical care, but it must meet more than the needs of the medical, nursing, and all other departments in the hospital; it also must meet the external requirements imposed by billing services, the Centers for Medicare & Medicaid Services and other governmental regulatory bodies, The Joint Commission, and insurance agencies. Physicians need to be able to access data, place orders, and document records, and they need software support for safety and medical decision making. Nurses and other clinical staff need to access documentation; there must be support for a closed-loop medication process and "the five rights." Billing, registration, lab, radiology, and other departments all need access to reports and data as well as careful integration with all other services and departments throughout the hospital.

When picking a vendor, we need a clear appreciation of the features we require (or will soon require) so that we can compare those features with their costs (and with the costs of **not** installing those features). Unless we know our goals, we cannot measure value. Which vendor offers the most value and is affordable? The choice also depends on how much a hospital wants to do things its own way as opposed to the way things are done elsewhere. Some hospitals complain that "our vendor is making us do it their way instead of our way," while other hospitals complain that the vendor "won't tell us the best way; they want us to reinvent the wheel." Some hospitals prefer to customize the design of the system; others prefer to have the vendor make design decisions. These conflicts parallel the differences between vendors:

- Some vendors offer systems that are "out of the box." The advantage is that one size fits all and you know exactly what you're getting. There are few bells and whistles, few decisions to make, and no options to consider. Upkeep is simple.
- Other vendors offer systems that are customizable. The advantage is that you can choose exactly the options you want, adapt the system to fit your needs, and adjust it as medicine (and the regulatory world) changes.

While there is no ideal system, there may be an ideal system for your particular hospital, one that fits not only your software needs but also your preference for simplicity versus flexibility. When evaluating a vendor, make sure you understand what you expect it to deliver: a completely designed system that offers no customization or a system that can be configured to fit your individual hospital. Should it be a turnkey system that has no options (but may be easier to design and install) or a customizable system that has many options (but may require more work to design and install)?

Site Visits: *Caveat Emptor*

Be careful of your site visits to other hospitals that use your proposed vendor. The vendor has carefully chosen the hospitals as its best examples, and you are there to evaluate the vendor, not the hospitals. Sophisticated CEOs would never buy a car because of the sexy person driving it in the advertisement; they need to be equally careful not to select a vendor because of the impressive hospital "driving" the system. Site visits are useful but misleading: You rarely see problems, and it's easy to see an institution you want to emulate rather than an EHR system that works.

WHO ARE THE VENDORS?

The three largest vendors are Cerner, Epic, and Eclipsys, but this statement is equivocal; it reflects only vendors in the US market, does not define *largest*, and is a static assessment rather than a reflection of trends. Moreover, it does not mention quality, the potential return on investment for a hospital using one of the three vendors, or the vendors' ability to install quickly and provide future support. Caveats aside, it is accurate; these three vendors control the bulk of the US market and receive the highest satisfaction ratings.

And the Winner Is . . .

According to Black Book Rankings (2012), a division of Brown-Wilson Group and an unbiased source of market research, the following are top-ranked EHR vendors:

- Top-ranked inpatient hospital EHR vendor—chains and IDN software vendors: Cerner
- Top-ranked inpatient EHR vendor—small and rural hospitals (fewer than 100 beds): CPSI
- Top-ranked acute care EHR software vendor—community hospitals (101 to 250 beds): Cerner
- Top-ranked acute care EHR software vendor—large medical centers / hospitals (more than 250 beds): GE Healthcare
- Top-ranked inpatient emergency department EHR software vendor: Picis

---

Curiously, two of the three vendors both claim to be the largest, but this definition depends on whether the measure is the number of hospitals (Cerner) or the number of physicians (Epic) currently using their systems. Epic has a reputation of going for (a few) large clients, whereas Cerner goes for (many) smaller hospitals with fewer physicians on staff. In the past, some smaller hospitals complained that Epic wouldn't consider them as a client. As one CEO commented, "Epic won't take you on unless you're big," although this situation appears to be changing. After the big three, several midsize vendors are worth noting, including Meditech, McKesson, CPSI, GE Healthcare, Siemens, Quadramed, Healthland, and HMS. Some of these vendors (e.g., CPSI) have a higher market share of small community hospitals than do the big three. All have their own strengths and adherents. The three major vendors receive mixed reviews from physicians; no matter the system, some physicians will hate it and others will love it.

Incidentally, the wide variation in users' love/hatred for a particular system equally applies to the one major noncommercial system in use in the United States: the military hospital system, commonly referred to as the VA (Veterans Administration) system. This system is not used commercially, so it will not be discussed further in this book.

WHICH VENDOR DO CLINICAL STAFFS LIKE BEST?

Whatever the commercial system—Cerner, Epic, Eclipsys, or another—reviews are mixed; there is no consensus on which system is best for all clinical care. The one curious consistency is that in general, the longer physicians use a system, the more they tend to like it. High ratings correlate with both the length of time a system has been in use and the "penetration" of the system in the hospital. As a system becomes exclusive in all parts of a hospital (i.e., achieves higher penetration), it becomes more highly rated by the hospital's employees, including the physician staff.

In short, the longer you use it and the more places you see it, the more you like it.

Whether physicians like a system or not has slowly become less of an issue for hospitals. There are three reasons for this shift:

1. Physicians are getting used to the idea that everyone is going to be using an EHR of some sort, whether they like it or not (so grumbling has diminished over the past decade).
2. The systems are gradually improving. They are more user-friendly, require less staff training, and are easier to customize.
3. Physicians understand that implementation of an EHR is essential to meeting meaningful-use criteria and hence ultimately affects their hospital's income.

INITIAL AND LONG-TERM VENDOR SUPPORT

Until recently, hospitals looked at traditional criteria when judging a vendor: cost, value, physician adoption, and so forth. Now, a major criterion is whether a vendor can install a system fast enough to meet meaningful-use criteria.

In this regard, the big-three vendors are ranked as more likely to be able to install and support their systems for most of their customers in time to meet the criteria, while the smaller vendors are generally thought to be less dependable in this regard, although no known data exist to support or disprove these opinions. After the big three, Meditech and McKesson have newer, updated software but will need to markedly increase their past rates of installation if their customers are going to achieve the criteria in time.

Post-installation, the vendor's ability to support the client's current installation and future updates is also important. Meeting deadlines imposed by the American Recovery & Reinvestment Act (e.g., meaningful use) is one thing; the ability to foresee and meet future deadlines is another. While government regulation is a major concern and while this concern projects forward into a future in which the only certainty is that the regulatory burden will increase, a great number of other changes are also probably in store for hospitals. While most hospitals will be electronic in a matter of years, new features and new abilities are already foreseen and will continue to alter the market.

NICHES DISAPPEAR, BUT TECHNOLOGY FILLS THE GAP

Not only is a good system able to communicate with other systems and other facilities; it also is able to accommodate *widgets:* applications that are not part of the original vendor's system but have capabilities that are valuable to particular users. Applications designed by individual physicians, nurses, and others who work independently of the software vendor will markedly increase the utility and flexibility of the vendor's interface. Medical widgets will become a day-to-day, critical part of clinical workflow; each specialty will have its own collection of tools to use to get more done, and to get it done more quickly, easily, and reliably than is currently the case. While issues of licensing, safety, compatibility, and confidentiality are certain to arise, widgets' potential is great, and they already are being incorporated into current systems.

Natural language systems will be taking word recognition programs to the next level by parsing the grammar and synonyms used in medical documentation and returning to dictation as a useful form of documentation. The use of natural language systems will enable the computer to pull billing information and mine data directly from a physician's dictation as well as provide clinical decision support and enforce regulatory compliance in real time during dictation. Several vendors already are using natural language engines to acquire billing information and partnering with Dragon Systems to develop language systems for physician order entry and other functions. Video documentation; multiple media inputs; and systems offering dynamic differential diagnosis

Proof of Benefit

A recent report published by The Advisory Board Company and HIMSS Analytics (2012) indicates that advanced users of EHRs, both healthcare systems and individual hospitals, realized substantial clinical quality, operational efficiency, and patient safety benefits. In addition to these clinical and patient benefits, hospitals reported achieving a number of other operational and administrative benefits, including the following:

Reported Benefit	Percentage Response
Reduced order turnaround times	76
Improved drug order-to-administration time	73
Decreased cost of paper forms	67
Improved charge capture	64
Decreased transcription costs	61
Reduced duplicate lab testing	58
Reduced antibiotic start times	58
Improved documentation quality	55
Improved quality of coding	46
Reduced health information management/ medical records staffing	42
Improved reimbursement	42
Reduced payment denials	39
Pharmacist time savings	33
Reduced drug use or cost	30
Reduced clinical costs	24
Reduced length of stay	18
Nursing staff time savings	15
Increased use of preventive care	12
Reduced staffing	9
Other	6
Don't know	3
We have not realized any additional benefit	3

and therapeutic suggestions in response to real-time changes in a patient's history, examinations, workups, or vital signs are only a few of the upcoming changes we are likely to see in newer systems over the next several years. When evaluating a vendor, ask how committed it is to future clinical technologies, or you may find yourself committed to choosing another vendor.

KEY POINTS

- Define the scope of your specific needs, and choose your vendor accordingly.
- Can you work with the vendor as a **partner**?
- Can your clinical staff use the system easily?
- How much build or training does the system require?
- Can the vendor support you both now and in the future?
- Will the vendor be able to adapt to future technology and regulatory changes?

CHAPTER 3

Governance

There are some people who are born leaders.
But the best leaders work at it day in and day out.

—Kenneth Chenault

EFFECTIVE LEADERSHIP—like many important lessons—is simpler to explain than to implement. Good governance not only builds on committee and reporting structures that are definable and easy to duplicate; it also requires personal behaviors that are known (but ignored) and other personal characteristics that may be difficult to teach. To some extent, the born leader starts with such behaviors—characteristics that make it easy to lead—but these behaviors can be learned. The difficulty lies not so much in learning these behaviors as in the quotidian performance of these behaviors.

Understanding **how to be** a leader is not equivalent to **being** a leader.

While the bulk of this chapter is aimed specifically at the leadership required to implement and optimize computer systems in hospitals, the same issues (with the exception of changes to the specific committee structures required) pertain to hospital leadership in general and, indeed, to leadership in any human endeavor.

LEADERSHIP: EFFECTIVE CHARACTERISTICS

There is a tendency to characterize leaders as charismatic, tall, attractive, intelligent, and a host of other—largely irrelevant and superficial—qualities. Perhaps these factors correlate with leadership, but even at best they merely correlate with deeper characteristics, imperfectly observed, that are the essence of leadership. Charisma is the reflection of critical behaviors that are valued by those you lead, including honesty, reliability, and responsibility. Height is often perceived from social presence rather than physical stature, and the reality is often startling. Good looks are often our perception of the personality animating an individual's facial expressions, combined with grooming and an ability to be at ease in social settings. Intelligence in this context is almost always more **social** intelligence than other types of intelligence. At best, these characteristics can be markers of leadership but are not leadership per se, just as common clinical biomarkers correlate with the pathology of a disease but are not the disease itself.

Good leaders may occasionally be born, but there is no special gene for leadership. Leaders possess a group of characteristics that we value, and many of those characteristics can be not only defined but also taught. In looking at these characteristics, we must distinguish what is **simple** from what is **easy**. When I give a test of ethics to executive candidates, the principles may be simple and getting a perfect grade may even be easy, but **performing** ethically is another matter and may not be easy at all. Likewise, defining the principles of leadership may be simple in that the rules are simply defined, but an effort is required to carry out those behaviors. They may be easy in the sense that the actions are trivial, but leaders must be committed to them and willing to take the social or political risks these "simple" actions may incur.

Let's consider examples of good leadership in several disparate contexts, including being a good parent and a good committee chair, as well as what prevents leadership behavior.

The Two-and-a-Half Problem

A wife once asked her husband why their children obeyed him but not her. The cause, he said, was the "two-and-a-half problem."

He would count to three, while she would count "one, two, two-and-a-half," progressively closing in on three but never getting to three. The children knew their father would reach three and invoke whatever consequences were incumbent on the statement; their mother would never reach the limit and therefore could safely be ignored. She was, in some sense, reliably unreliable.

Put more simply and far less charitably, she was being dishonest.

Much of day-to-day behavior is exactly the same: We strenuously defend our honesty and reliability, but our actual behavior—in small, daily, often unnoticed actions—speaks otherwise. We understand the principle, but we fail to act on it and often don't recognize what we are doing as we routinely undercut our leadership.

The principle here is predictability, although it can be looked at as either honesty or reliability. A logical child infers that a person counting to two-and-a-half will never invoke consequences, and the same inference is made in leadership settings. If I, as a CEO, threaten to cancel a physician's staff privileges unless he uses CPOE and then don't carry through on this action, I must expect my medical staff to discount me on future occasions. Even the most logical, unemotional physician will infer that my words are unrelated to my actions and will act accordingly. Not only have I undercut my credibility (acted dishonestly)—I have undercut my ability to lead.

Ethics: A Practical Leadership Tool

The same problem—with the same costs—often occurs in our behavior with regard to ethics. Few of us would fail a corporate test of ethics, and while we may not perceive our ethical breaches, those around us are acutely aware—and deeply critical of us—when our behaviors reveal our unethical habits. Leadership does not depend on tests of honesty, ethics, diversity, knowledge, or other measures; it depends on our day-to-day behavior. We judge those around us—and particularly leaders—from their small actions rather than from their grand gestures. Leaders strive to recognize and correct their inconsistencies, not merely in what they say on an exam or in a formal talk but in what they do every day, everywhere, and in every action. Effective communication involves a parallel: The key is not in what you say but in what others understand. In leadership, the critical feature is not your internal justifications but how others interpret your behavior.

Responsibility is not just an **internal** characteristic; it is also an **interpersonal** characteristic: A good leader is perceived as responsible, and the leader expects others to be responsible. The need for honesty, ethics, and responsibility may be obvious, yet these behaviors are uncommon; they are given lip service, but often little more. Their basic utility as characteristics of leadership rather than unrealistic ideals often goes unrecognized as having concrete benefits. In almost all contexts, bad leadership consists of not following obvious strategies.

Good leadership consists largely of doing the obvious.

KEY LEADERSHIP STRATEGIES

In defining responsibility and its failure, particularly in the case of medical IT projects, we emphasize three key strategies: enforcing deadlines, defining and communicating agendas, and tasking.

Deadlines

Deadlines are not advisory; they are disasters waiting to happen. Medical IT projects are heavily interdependent, relying on close coordination between most clinical departments, as well as the IT department, project management, key physicians, and the executive suite. When a deadline is pushed back or missed, it becomes a case of "for want of a nail, a kingdom was lost."

When one person or one group misses a deadline, the next person is delayed, and the result cascades into a potential avalanche of failure. All deadlines mesh; one error has ramifications well beyond the obvious. In one hospital, a group "cleaning up" the orderables catalog was sorry it had "gotten behind," but it had little understanding of the consequences of being behind. Not only were the order sets not ready (because the catalog wasn't available); the delay made testing and training impossible (train with what orderables and what order sets?), causing the conversion date to be postponed several months. And there were other consequences. The budget was badly undermined because the hospital was unable to readjust schedules to backfill during the altered training dates and the conversion, the vendor and the consulting group were unable to meet the new conversion dates, and the project went well over budget. For want of an orderables catalog, a conversion was lost—and almost a hospital as well.

Knowing that the word *deadline* can quickly become accurate, a good leader ensures that deadlines are kept.

Agendas

Agendas—and committee strategies in general—are a boring aspect of corporate structure, but like deadlines, they are a critical aspect of good leadership. In well-run corporate structures, agendas have several common characteristics:

- Agendas are defined ahead of time and communicated to everyone.
- Meetings begin on time, every time; they likewise end on time, every time.
- Individuals are assigned responsibility for items on the agenda.
- Time limits are defined (or well understood) for each agenda item.
- A default or standard agenda provides structure and prevents omissions.
- Decisions are made and future actions are well defined.

These "little things"—which are not truly little at all—are often underestimated or even ignored, but these strategies are necessary to success. In the best hospitals, they are automatic, a part of hospital culture; in successful hospitals, they may or may not be automatic, but they are enforced.

Agendas need to be defined and communicated. Defining and communicating an agenda ahead of time prepares committee members for the meeting or—in the negative case—helps them recognize when their presence is unnecessary and their time would be wasted if they attended. Letting members know what to expect ahead of time increases the credibility (the honesty) of the committee and its goals. Requiring physicians (or others) to come to a meeting in which they are not needed (or even referred to) is a sure way to make attendance flag and to undercut the goals of the committee.

Every meeting needs reliable time limits. Meetings should have defined beginnings and endings. Members who arrive on time should be rewarded, not punished. When a committee chair suggests that on-time members "wait just a few minutes for the others," he ensures that they will consider being tardy for the next meeting and also ensures that those who are tardy will realize that they can be even more tardy. This scenario is a classic case of the two-and-a-half problem in a committee venue.

Each agenda item needs an owner. Not only should agenda items each be **assigned to an individual**; the person also needs to be aware of his responsibility ahead of time. In the extreme case, every agenda item might be the responsibility of the chair or the committee secretary, but regardless, responsibility must be assigned and overt.

Each agenda item needs a time limit. Time limits may occasionally be flexible at the discretion of the chair or at the consensus of the committee members, but once again there is an element of the two-and-a-half problem. If I know that I can ramble on about my pet peeve during the meeting, others will wonder why they

---

Sample Agenda

The following list is a sample standing agenda from an actual hospital's physician advisory group:

- Adoption
- Communication
- System design
- Order sets
- Workflow
- Technical
- Testing
- Outcome measures
- Training
- Conversion readiness

A time (e.g., five minutes) and an owner (e.g., chief medical information officer [CMIO]) are assigned to each item for each meeting.

---

attended and wasted their time. Each agenda item needs a time window, and it is the responsibility of the chair or the secretary to watch the time and enforce closure, either by moving on to the next item or by voting on an action.

Have a standard agenda. Every useful committee has a purpose. Successful committees use that purpose to define a standard or default agenda that includes items addressed in almost every meeting. Standing agendas ensure that important items are not overlooked by providing a "tickler" or a holding place for each of them.

Make decisions clearly and define tasking. The hallmark of an ineffectual committee is to avoid decisions that can (and must) be made or to make decisions without instituting action. Tasking is the linchpin of executive behavior.

Tasking

Far and away the most common failure—and the most important issue in committee leadership—is tasking behavior. Too often, a committee considers an action (e.g., "Let's see what our legal counsel thinks of this policy") and the vote carries, but there is a complete lack of tasking, and then everyone wonders why the next meeting shows no progress has been made. Decision is useless without action; action requires clear tasking with follow-up.

Effective committee behavior depends on five tasking components:

1. What task must be performed?
2. Who must perform the task?
3. When is the deadline for the task?
4. How is the task to be accomplished?
5. Where does oversight of the task reside?

In the example given earlier (i.e., "Let's see what our legal counsel thinks of this policy"), the tasking might be as follows:

- **What:** Contact the hospital legal counsel and request an opinion.
- **Who:** John, the CMIO of the hospital, will contact the counsel.
- **When:** John will receive the counsel's answer by Tuesday at 10 a.m.
- **How:** Ask the hospital counsel for a verbal opinion and write it up.
- **Where:** John will e-mail the result to Mary, the committee chair.

In every task, **with no exception**, these aspects must—in one form or another—be clearly understood and preferably spelled out precisely in every committee meeting. There is no task so inconsequential that it can be left to an undefined "someone" who will do

---

Point to Remember

Tasking behavior is necessary not only to committee action but equally so elsewhere in the hospital. Medical codes can be confusing and stressful, and they become all the more so when a physician gives an un-tasked order:

"Someone give the patient a milligram of epi!"

Unless the physician assigns the task to an individual, the physician risks not having it administered or having it administered twice. Tasking behavior provides clarity:

"Mary, please give the patient a milligram of epi, stat."

Tasking not only is good manners and essential to keeping codes organized; it also encourages similar organized and appropriate behavior among the rest of the medical team. This same behavior is required for a committee to fulfill an executive role.

Tasking Behaviors

For any task, defining
  What, Who, When, How, Where = Effective Outcome.

"something" at "sometime" and so forth. Committees that don't have defined tasking behaviors rapidly become ineffectual and contribute to the failure of any project. The responsibility lies with the chair, but the culture of an effective hospital supports tasking behaviors and often requires them. Tasking cannot be wishful thinking; it demands that follow-through be defined and enforced.

Useful Committee Strategies

Many organizations have discovered other, less crucial strategic tools to use in a committee structure. They include (1) requiring that all arguments be confined to a subcommittee charged with making a specific recommendation and (2) ranking priorities while requiring that all politicking for such priorities be forbidden within the committee meeting and restricted to outside discussion.

Restricting Arguments to a Subcommittee

Many large, unwieldy committees have discovered the value of subcommittees yet missed an opportunity to use them to streamline fact gathering, discussion, and voting. While the main committee is responsible for the final executive vote, there is no reason the first two stages—fact gathering and discussion—cannot be pared off to a subcommittee. This strategy is often followed, if a bit informally, and produces efficient results. In its best form, the committee tasks the subcommittee to gather facts, discuss the options, and specify a recommended action. (The key is to prevent these three behaviors from recurring in the main committee.) The main committee hears the recommendation and the rationale for it, clarifies any questions of fact, and then votes on the subcommittee's recommendation. If the vote carries, the recommendation becomes action; if the vote fails, the issue goes back to the subcommittee for reconsideration.

The main committee does not permit discussion or arguments about alternatives, except to clarify facts; as stated earlier, politicking and presentation of opinions are not permitted. This rule is critical and must be enforced. It vests responsibility for a clear recommendation to the subcommittee (although executive responsibility still resides with the main committee) and ensures the main committee is executive, not argumentative. The time savings can be enormous.

Restricting Arguments to Personal Time

The second technique is used to establish priorities (e.g., financial priorities for an institution) without wasting committee time arguing about them. Suppose, for example, that a hospital can fund only a specific capital budget for the next fiscal year. The committee members are given a complete list of all potential capital projects and are invited to list (privately) their own perceived priorities. They are told that their lists will be combined and that their priorities will be averaged to create a final list of hospital priorities for the next fiscal year. The hospital will fund the projects, moving down the list until the available budget is exhausted. No further projects will then be funded, no matter how important they may be to any particular committee member, nor will any discussion of those relative priorities be tolerated within the committee. Every member of the committee, however, should feel free (indeed, is encouraged) to buttonhole other committee members outside of the meeting and get them to change their list of priorities. If this politicking changes the combined master list of priorities, so be it. This technique can be adapted to many situations and can be invaluable, as long as the chair (who is enforcing this technique) takes care to prevent cabals from forming and marginalizing specific committee members who are legitimately representing the real needs of a specific hospital department or service.

LEADERSHIP: EFFECTIVE STRUCTURES

Prior to beginning any project, hospitals already have in place a governance structure that defines responsibility and controls resources. The *implementation* phase (e.g., beginning the use of CPOE) requires specific changes to be made to that governance structure. Those changes are ingrained and become the standard mode of business during the *optimization* phase.

It would be easy—but misleading—to infer that the committee and personnel required for a project are merely grafted onto the hospital's "real" governance as temporary or negligible accessories. This misconception results from the notion that clinical IT projects are just a matter of adding software and hardware to the current clinical landscape. In reality, these projects profoundly alter clinical practice, hospital culture, and the governance structure of a hospital, and the changes are useful, predictable, and permanent. The perception that this alteration is—at least initially in certain cases—inconsequential can lead to project failure and problems for hospital leadership.

In this regard, the most obvious change in the past decade has been the addition of the CMIO to the executive suite of most hospitals. This addition has posed uncertainties that are still far from resolved. The underlying and often unanswered (or even unrecognized) question is—at least with regard to clinical IT—*Who's running the show?* In many conservative hospitals, the answer has been the IT department, as embodied in the CIO. In others, the answer has changed: The clinical staff are running the show, and the system is ultimately under the control of the CMIO—a difference that reflects the increasing emphasis on the **clinical** nature of current IT systems; IT isn't "just computers." While responsibility and reporting order (more CMIOs reporting directly to the CEO) are gradually shifting, defining this aspect of hospital governance remains problematic and in flux. What is clear is that clinical input and direction remain crucial and that most hospitals now designate a CMIO as part of their governance structure, however reporting order may be defined.

Governance for Implementation

Implementations generally are governed by a combined leadership structure encompassing hospital administration (usually with at least one key player from the C-suite), the clinical staff (e.g., physicians and nurses, perhaps represented by the CMO and CNO), the project manager, the IT department, the vendor, and other key players (e.g., pharmacy) as required. Success depends not just on getting physicians involved but also on having a healthy administrative culture (evaluation of leadership is discussed later in this chapter).

The least common denominator is to have a governance "tree" that includes an executive committee, a project committee, and a clinical committee (see Exhibits 3.1 and 3.2). Depending on the size and previous political structures of the hospital, these committees are often created *de novo*, largely independent (but cognizant) of previous clinical committee structures, such as the medical executive committee and the pharmacy and therapeutics committee.

Exhibit 3.1: Governance Tree

Members	Committee	Concern
C-suite	Executive steering	Hospital success
CMIO, CIO, vendor, etc.	Project steering	Project success
MDs, RNs, pharmacy	Clinical steering	Clinical success

Exhibit 3.2: Governance Committee Structure

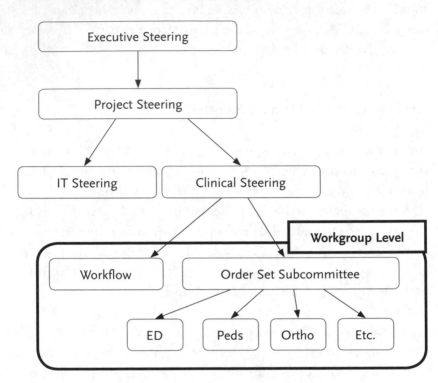

The **executive steering committee** is responsible for ensuring that the project meets the long-term needs of the hospital and consists of hospital members, generally the C-suite or executive sponsors (e.g., CFO, COO, CMO, CNO). This group makes all high-level decisions, especially those with profound policy, legal, or financial ramifications.

The **project steering committee** is responsible for project success. It includes hospital members and may include members (even voting members) of the vendor or third-party consultants, particularly a project manager. Also part of the committee are members who are neither executive nor clinical but directly responsible for the actual hardware and software, including the CIO (who may also be

Executive Steering Committee

Membership includes

- an executive sponsor,
- a project manager (often including the vendor), and
- hospital officers (CIO, CMO, CNO, CMIO).

Responsibilities include

- aligning business objectives with the hospital vision,
- supervision of the project team,
- supervision of the physician advisory committee, and
- overcoming operational obstacles that require high-level action.

Project Steering Committee

Membership includes

- the CIO and other executive members as appropriate;
- project managers (including the vendor);
- the CMIO, CMO, and CNO, as appropriate;
- the hospital IT department; and
- IT architects and build personnel.

Responsibilities include

- oversight of all project timelines and budget;
- supervision of all project personnel;
- coordination and oversight of clinical and IT committees; and
- oversight of build, installation, domains, hardware updates, and so forth.

on the executive committee) and other IT personnel, such as system architects and programmers. In many ways, this committee is the project itself: It maintains deadlines, has responsibility for project outcomes, oversees all working groups (both technical and clinical), and coordinates system testing, user training, and so forth. In well-run projects, this committee exemplifies a good, balanced working relationship between the hospital, the vendor, and (if present) the third-party consultant. It is responsible **to** the executive committee and **for** the clinical and technical working groups.

The **clinical steering committee** is responsible for clinical success. This committee is often synonymous with a physician advisory group (PAG), physician advisory committee (PAC), or similar aggregations. If they are not synonymous, the PAG (or PAC) reports directly to the clinical steering committee. The clinical steering committee (or if separate, the PAG or PAC) is responsible for evaluating

---

Clinical Steering Committee

Membership includes

- the CMIO or a physician champion (chair),
- physicians from major stakeholder groups,
- a nursing representative (e.g., CNO),
- the CIO (may not be a voting member), and
- a physician consultant (vendor).

Responsibilities include

- review of all content, especially order sets;
- review of all alerts and rules;
- review of all relevant policies and procedures;
- review of workflows (i.e., process issues);
- oversight of departmental working groups;
- serving as a clinical resource for the project; and
- communication with clinical personnel.

---

and recommending changes to the clinical policies (the purview of the medical executive committee), reviewing and defining acceptable workflows (for all clinical staff), and defining and maintaining software tools, such as order sets, alerts, standing orders, and clinical advisory systems. This committee, chaired by the physician leader, includes medical staff (especially physician champions) as well as nursing and pharmacy representatives. While the core membership is clinical, nonclinical (and often nonvoting) members (e.g., system analysts, project manager) are often useful resources for this committee. The project manager might be responsible for preparation of meeting materials, and the membership includes (often as nonvoting members) representation from the IT department and the vendor to clarify issues related to the design and build of the system. Although the clinical steering committee technically is "under" the project steering committee, its responsibilities and reporting take on an increasingly critical and executive nature as most projects progress to fruition. This evolution should be expected; after the implementation, this committee has long-term responsibility for system oversight and optimization. The implementation project ends, but the **rationale** for that implementation was clinical, and clinical needs remain central to the hospital. The most obvious part of this permanent responsibility is the maintenance and updating of order sets and alerts.

Another committee underlying the project steering committee is the **IT steering committee**. This group is responsible for installing the hardware and software and ensuring they support the clinical goals of the system. The committee initially includes a portion of the hospital's IT services staff and vendor experts. As the project progresses—especially after implementation—the vendor members become superfluous (one hopes) and the IT steering committee merges back into the day-to-day workings of the hospital's IT department.

Under the clinical steering committee (or if separate from the clinical steering committee, the PAG or PAC) are the working clinical committees. The most obvious subgroup is the **order set**

committee. This working (rather than executive) group is responsible for defining and enforcing a style and nomenclature for the hospital's order sets as well as ensuring that each specialty submits and/or reviews the initial order sets for the implementation. For example, this group might maintain a spreadsheet listing the 400 order sets that will be created, ensure that the orthopedic group submits its 20 order sets on time, and confirm that those 20 order sets follow the established format. The detailed working of this committee is discussed in Chapter 5.

Another "group" under the clinical steering committee is responsible for managing workflows. This responsibility generally is not assigned to a committee but rather to one (or a few) individuals. They are charged not only with understanding the current clinical workflows but also with defining exactly how the workflows must change upon implementation to achieve success and maintain safety. This work must be accomplished by—and is required for—the training phase prior to implementation.

Governance for Optimization

Optimization is the (optimistic) name given to the process that ensues after a hospital has implemented a system. In this phase, hospitals should focus not only on optimizing the current system but also on maintaining the clinical relevance and accuracy of the catalog, order sets, alerts, and other clinical tools. Moreover, not only do systems change and improve, necessitating active participation by hospital governance; even the **intent** of such systems changes. Hospitals already are using their systems for more than merely placing orders and shaping clinical judgment by reference to outside sources of expertise; they also are mining their own clinical data to improve day-to-day clinical actions.

The governance structure necessary to long-term system usage (i.e., optimization) is little different from a traditional hospital governance structure. Successful hospitals commonly (indeed, almost universally) maintain the committee structure charged with oversight of clinical IT. This committee, generally chaired by the CMIO of the hospital, is predominantly clinical in composition. While physicians are the plurality, nurses, pharmacists, and other stakeholders are often present, including IT representatives. This committee almost always grows directly out of either the clinical steering committee or the PAG/PAC. The reporting structures vary but generally encompass the C-suite and/or the hospital's medical executive committee.

The aim of this group is no longer to direct the implementation of IT but to optimize the technology to support efficient and safe clinical care. The emphasis is not on making decisions about a new and largely unknown system but rather on improving a known system by optimizing options, order sets, and clinical workflows. Optimization often involves rethinking old decisions in the light of experience. The system must be kept up to date and improved even in the unlikely event that clinical users are perfectly happy with the system as it stands. Not only do regulatory requirements change; so does clinical practice, and it behooves the hospital to adjust its system, its order sets, and its workflows to remain in sync with changing circumstances.

Governance for Future Changes

Both hardware (e.g., tablets, smartphones) and software are continually changing. Until now, changes to software largely have been incremental as vendors tweaked and added features to their products. As discussed in later chapters, however, at least two incoming waves of change will require hospitals to actively evaluate and respond. The first is the advent of a plethora of widgets, add-ons, and overlays that will markedly affect how systems are used. The second is the upcoming shift from manual to verbal input for those systems.

The advent of small programs that can be separately purchased and that will reside "on top of" current systems will require a diffusion of governance in the hospital. A decade ago, each department might purchase a niche system to meet its specific needs (e.g., labor and delivery, ED). A decade from now, each department—while still part of the institution-wide system—will likely have specific add-on programs that will once again meet its specific needs. These changes will be welcome and will support better and more efficient care if they are vetted and evaluated to coordinate with the needs of other departments. Departments will need to evaluate add-ons for their ability to meet their specific clinical needs; hospital governance will need to evaluate add-ons for their ability to meet the system needs of the hospital. While hospital-wide governance will remain viable and necessary, there will be a gradual shift toward more diffuse input and evaluation by hospital departments. To remain effective and competitive, a good hospital will anticipate this change and incorporate it into its planning.

The upcoming shift to verbal input will affect both order entry and documentation. This change is already in progress via word recognition programs, such as Dragon Nuance, which is used either as a stand-alone application or in conjunction with template-driven electronic documentation. The next step is free-form verbal documentation that is capable of using verbal macros, reminding physicians and nurses of missing components "on the fly" as they document, and extracting billing data without requiring that the documenter have any specific knowledge of billing (as opposed to medical) coding information. This technology promises to improve the efficiency of clinical documentation while also improving regulatory, billing, and legal outcomes and not requiring that the documenter be an expert in any of these "nonclinical" areas. Reality, however, may diverge from this promise. The role of hospital governance—in regard to verbal order entry and verbal documentation—will be to continue to evaluate the technology and balance the disparate clinical and nonclinical needs of the hospital.

Outsourcing Governance

Two factors have provided impetus for an increasing number of hospitals to outsource their medical IT needs. The first factor is the specialized nature of hospital information systems; many smaller hospitals cannot afford to find, train, and/or maintain such specialized personnel and systems. The second factor is the transition in the vendor market from implementations toward consulting and optimization.

Consider the first issue: the hospital perspective. Until recently, few hospitals had experience with implementing medical software. The expertise was supplied by the vendor, a third-party consulting team, or both. In addition, while many hospitals maintained their own hardware (i.e., servers) and software, it was tempting to farm out fulfillment of reliability, rapid access, and software maintenance requirements to a remote hosting organization (RHO), especially given the rapidly changing technology base. While outsourcing incurred obvious costs, it also cut the costs of in-house technical personnel and upgrades while guaranteeing reliability.

The second issue derives from the vendor market. While the market for implementation (particularly in the United States) is enormous (as hospitals respond to regulatory needs), and while vendors' attempts to meet this demand have prompted huge hiring increases, most vendors anticipate that this market will decline markedly in the next several years. However, the need for consultants to optimize, manage, and update systems after implementation is likely to increase. Anticipating this trend, many vendors are moving (or planning to move) into the medical IT governance market, specifically by serving not only as RHOs for hospitals (as described in the previous paragraph) but also as CMIOs and by providing IT support.

The short-term (next decade) market trend is clear: More and more hospitals will outsource governance of their medical IT. Whether this trend will continue long term or whether hospitals will find themselves capable of managing their own internal needs more cheaply and efficiently is unclear.

Common Threads in Governance

In every hospital implementing a medical IT system, a number of issues are ubiquitous. Such issues carry a common theme: the tension between those planning the system and those using the system. This theme surfaces in a number of specific problems all hospitals have, including the issues of risk versus workflow, up-front work versus user work, and standardization versus customization, and in the overarching issues arising from policies and procedures.

The issue of risk versus workflow is common to almost every governance decision. For example, many systems enable a physician to open multiple patient charts simultaneously. If a hospital limits the user to a single chart at a time, it may lower patient risk (but see later chapters for a more sophisticated evaluation of such risks), but this restriction will impede workflow: Delivery of patient care will become slower. As another example, if a hospital requires that nurses have a second nurse witness and electronically sign the chart for certain high-risk drugs, it may decrease the risk of drug errors, but this requirement will similarly affect workflow: Patient care will be delivered more slowly. This issue—risk versus workflow—arises in almost every decision, committee, and governance discussion during system implementation and design. We can almost never decrease risk without incurring some cost, usually a negative effect on workflow. The right question is not "Should we lower risk?" but "Does the lower risk justify the costs to patient care?" Answering that question correctly requires thought and sophistication, not a knee-jerk response.

Up-front work versus user work is a classic case of an "unfunded mandate." In this type of decision, project managers opt to forego work on the system (e.g., weeding out inappropriate drug routes from a long drop-down list for each medication) without considering that the user incurs an unfunded mandate to their time as a result: The user is forced to weed through the long, inappropriate drop-down list of drug routes for every drug, every patient, every day. Overall, this extra effort markedly increases the costs of patient care: Physicians and nurses cannot see as many patients, patients receive slower care, and the risk of errors goes up. Because these costs are spread out—each drug order becomes "only" several seconds longer—they are less visible to the planners and do not show as line item costs to the project budget. Nonetheless, all the project managers have done is shifted the up-front work (and cost) to the user, and the overall cost of the system is markedly increased, not decreased.

Standardization versus customization is another recurrent theme with good arguments for each position. In industrial planning, variance is always detrimental. The complexity of medicine, particularly the complexity of genetic variance and human interaction, forces a certain amount of variance into patient care that cannot always be swept away. Moreover, we can anticipate innovation and improvement in medical care, so it would be detrimental if we were to standardize last year's medicine and prevent next year's advances. On the other hand, in day-to-day medicine, a certain amount of care is known to be ineffective, expensive, and unnecessary. The most appropriate way of balancing standardization and customization—at least in most hospitals and in most medical IT systems—is not to totally prevent variance but to erect partial barriers to variance. In the case of order sets, we do not forbid the use of nonstandard care but rather make it easy to provide standard care and harder to provide nonstandard care. Physicians who want to order a more expensive and putatively less effective drug can do so, but they have to go through more effort, jump through hoops, and surmount obstacles to do so. Hospitals and medical IT systems vary—some require almost full standardization of all care, while others permit almost any customization—but however a particular hospital balances these two needs, this issue is ubiquitous.

These issues lie behind almost every committee meeting and every decision. The formal arena in which these issues play out is that of policy-and-procedure decisions. Such issues are defined in the medical bylaws and staff regulations of every hospital. Do we require CPOE? Do we require electronic documentation? Do we allow copy-forward functions in our documentation? These issues and others like them cause tension between system planners and clinical users. System planners know that there are preventable errors and want to standardize; clinical users know that there is a certain amount of intrinsic variance and want to customize. If we never permit exceptions or variation, we incur significant costs and risks to patient care. If we allow free rein, we equally incur significant costs and risks to patient care.

Rarely are any of these complex issues solved by recourse to a single-minded, simple policy. Risks can never be reduced to zero,

Real-Life Examples

Case 1

A hospital in the greater New York City area initially forbade verbal orders and required physicians to place all orders via computer. There were **no** exceptions. In doing so, it hobbled emergent patient care: All medical codes became slower because stat medications had to be entered into a computer, thereby almost doubling the time it took to administer medications during codes. Likewise, when physicians were scrubbed in surgery, they were not permitted to give verbal orders for pain medications; the result was increased patient suffering and delayed treatment. The no-exceptions policy was later modified to permit the exceptions observed by most hospitals: Physicians were permitted to give verbal orders in the case of codes, when they were scrubbed, and so forth.

Case 2

A hospital in Louisiana required physicians to enter all orders via computer; no verbal orders were permitted. In one case, a physician who was at her child's soccer game was called for a pain medication order and the nurse refused to take a verbal order, demanding that the physician leave her child at the game and find a computer to enter the order. Later, the physicians were found to be actively avoiding the nurses during lunch because the nurses would not only ask for orders but, again, demand that the physicians find and log on to a computer to place the order rather than finish their meal. As a result, patients' pain medication orders were delayed. Eventually, the policy of no verbal orders was modified to permit appropriate leeway and improve the efficiency of patient care.

and risk prevention is always a trade-off. Moreover, software may be used to shape behavior (by raising or lowering obstacles to specific behaviors), but software cannot be used to prevent bad behavior. Whenever we try to bar a specific bad behavior, we invariably end up punishing all physicians for the poor practices of a handful, and do so at a significant cost.

The trade-off between risk and workflow is never one-way.

EVALUATING LEADERSHIP

Consulting groups often recommend that hospitals have their leadership evaluated prior to implementing a medical information system. On its face, this recommendation is eminently reasonable and probably effective, but there are two practical caveats: (1) Is it cost-effective to do so, and (2) will those who most need help get help? The answers are (1) it depends and (2) (unfortunately) no.

The first is the question of whether the evaluation is a good return on investment. The answer is not simply a matter of finding a reputable consulting group with a good track record that can efficiently evaluate hospital leadership and provide valid, practical, specific advice on how to improve it. The catch here is the "how to improve it" part. Specifying how to improve leadership may be relatively simple, but instituting effective improvements may be difficult, in which case the evaluation may be right on the nose but not cost-effective. For example, many leadership problems are cultural—that is, widespread in the organization and difficult to change. Equally, the leadership problems might be the leaders. A recommendation to replace those who hired the leadership consultants is politically difficult to phrase and never acted on. In either case, recommendations may be accurate but ineffective.

The second caveat is that those most likely to seek evaluation are the least likely to need help with leadership skills. More important (and almost universally true), hospitals that scoff at outside evaluation are precisely those that have ineffective leadership.

There is an extremely high correlation between being a bad leader and being pig-headedly sure that you can't be a better one.

So, to those of you who are such good leaders that you would like to improve (which is why you are good leaders in the first place), the recommendation stands:

1. Find a reputable consulting group.
2. Have it evaluate your leadership.
3. Act on its recommendations for improvement.

KEY POINTS

- Good leadership consists largely of doing what most of us know **should** be done but don't actually do.
- Tasking behavior is **critical:** Define what, who, when, how, and where.
- The leadership structure for implementation evolves into a simpler, more clinical structure for optimization.
- Balance must be continuously maintained, and trade-offs made, between risk and workflow.

CHAPTER 4

Orderables and Catalogs

Never neglect details.

—*Colin Powell*

SUCCESS LIES IN details. In CPOE, the details are in the catalog and success is defined by the orderables it contains. When the orderables are badly done, outcomes will be at least as bad. Successful implementation of CPOE requires a thoughtful, workmanlike approach to the orderables and to the catalog as a whole.

In the world of the hospital, physicians order *orderables*; collectively, orderables form a *catalog*. There is no universal standard catalog of orderables for all hospitals. Orderables and catalogs differ between hospitals—even hospitals owned by the same chain—and vary over time. Some orderables are available in one hospital and not in another. One hospital might have access to cardiac catheterization, but another may not; one hospital can order a particular serology "in house," but another has to send it out.

LOCAL FORMULARIES, LOCAL CATALOGS

Every hospital has to build and maintain its own catalog. Drug formularies are a bit different; a hospital may import a generalized, commercially available formulary, but this formulary must be pared down and adjusted to fit the hospital's drug inventory. No hospital can carry every available drug. A hospital usually carries not only the drugs it believes to be effective but, because contract prices vary year to year, also those that are most cost-effective. In the case of statins, H2 blockers, certain antibiotics, and many other modern drugs, one hospital will carry one drug of each of these types, while another hospital will carry another drug of each of these same types. In each case, a hospital formulary must reflect not what is available in the market nationally but what is available in the hospital's own pharmacy locally. The same principle pertains to laboratory tests (some of which must be sent to outside labs), radiology exams, and every other category of orderable.

The major categories in a catalog are obvious: drugs, laboratory tests, and diagnostic procedures (largely radiology tests). A number of less obvious categories also are typically included: surgical, office, and dental procedures; patient care orders (e.g., vital signs); referrals and consults; diet orders; respiratory care orders; a host of specialty tests (e.g., cardiology, endoscopy, point of care); central supply; scheduling; admit, discharge, and transfer orders; and so forth. For example, in a large urban hospital in the Midwest, pharmacy orders compose the largest category (more than 5,000 orderables), followed by radiology and laboratory tests (more than 1,000 each). Excluding synonyms, the entire hospital catalog contains a total of 11,000 orderables.

CLEANING UP YOUR CATALOG

Every hospital has had—in some form—a catalog of orderables for decades prior to implementing CPOE. Hospital pharmacies often have already been using a computerized catalog long before physicians move from paper to computer entry of pharmacy orders.

Whenever the move occurs—and whether for drugs, labs, tests, or other orderables—it brings about changes. One positive change is that once the catalog is "cleaned up," it is easier to manage; we can edit, sort, update, and find our data quickly and efficiently.

Unfortunately, we are assuming that the data are accurate in the first place; hence, the need to clean up the catalog is one of the first steps in implementing a computer system in a modern hospital. Each drug, for example, needs to map to a modern drug catalog (e.g., Multum) along with the dose, form, route, frequency, and other details. It is not enough to carry Tylenol without mapping it not only to acetaminophen but also to the oral acetaminophen tablet (not the capsule and certainly not the rectal suppository or the oral liquid) and the 325 mg form of that tablet. This mapping enables the hospital to attach additional information, such as allergies and interactions, to that drug orderable in its catalog, all of which is necessary to modern clinical practice.

During an implementation, catalog cleanup is a prerequisite for much of the project. If we don't have a final catalog, it is impossible to finish designing and building order sets, impossible to use order sets or orderables, impossible to train users, and impossible to meet the conversion date. Catalog cleanup is not only a prerequisite to implementation: If the update is delayed, a project can literally stop completely. The catalog must be completed early and accurately; the project depends on it.

MEDICATION PROCESS TEAM

A surprising number of issues—naming conventions, medical policy, legal restrictions, billing concerns, and so forth—arise as we develop a catalog and how it is to be used. The majority (but by no means all) of these issues are related to medication orders. As a result, most projects have a meds process team devoted to this particular set of issues. Because the orderables and catalog are critical to the entire project, this team reports directly to the project steering committee. It usually maintains close contact with the physician advisory group and other clinical committees to avoid making decisions that might clash with clinical—as opposed to pharmacy—requirements. The team is generally run by a pharmacist and may include an IT analyst, a design architect (often from the vendor), and a clinical strategist or another person with a clinical perspective. The members of this team often overlap with the team that designs the order sets. The meds process team develops an accurate, clinically useful catalog of medication orderables (e.g., acetaminophen) and their attached medication sentences (e.g., capsule, oral, 325 mg). They build each orderable and test how it functions both within the catalog and within the order sets that use it. An orderable must trigger the correct tasks for nursing, pharmacy, lab, radiology, billing, and so forth.

NAMING ISSUES

Names determine ease of use. A poorly named orderable not only slows down physicians and nurses (and thus patient care) but also increases the risk of medical error.

Prior to CPOE, most hospital orderables were not named with regard to those who **placed** the order; they were named solely with regard to those who **performed** the order. In the case of radiology, for example, orderables were named by the radiology department in accordance with their internal needs, generally with an eye toward billing and always idiosyncratically relative to other hospitals' names for the same exams. The ward secretary filled the role of translator. When the clinical physician (as opposed to the radiologist) asked for a chest X-ray, the secretary translated this clinical order into a corresponding radiology order that often had a different—and unexpected—name for the same orderable. While the ordering physician wanted a *doppler*, the radiologist called this test a different name, such as *NV* (for *nonvascular*). This particular example, drawn from a large, nationwide hospital chain, was found on the first day of CPOE use and—because of the unexpected and nonintuitive name—caused an order normally placed in seconds to be delayed by 16 minutes (due to having to phone radiology and so forth). This name would not have been among the first dozen (indeed, the first thousand) guesses of any ordering physician. While the physicians came to understand the peculiar, nonclinical terminology, the same problem recurs every time the hospitals in this chain hire a new physician, eight years later.

Naming conventions should reflect the clinical conventions of the physicians placing the orders. Radiologists, serology lab techs, and blood bank nurses have every right to use their own nomenclature internally, but the physicians have to be able to locate the order if they are to place the order in the first place. No clinical physician has ever referred to a doppler study as an NV, nor is NV an intuitive choice. Newly hired attending physicians and new residents reasonably expect that nationally accepted, common clinical names—such as those used in their resident training, wherever the hospital—will serve as effective search terms in any hospital catalog. The rationale that "we've always called it that" is feckless and of no help to new physicians and residents who were trained elsewhere across the globe.

Examples of Inappropriate Orderable Names (from actual hospital catalogs)

Common Clinical Name	Example of Radiology Names
Chest X-ray	GD X-ray chest
	XR diag chest
	DXR chest
	DR cx-ray
Doppler	NV
	Vas study
	Spec ultrasound
	RAD dop
	RAD US

Synonyms

To establish naming conventions that reflect the widely accepted, standard usage of ordering physicians rather than the narrow usage of the departments performing the test or procedure, hospitals can use synonyms.

Most catalogs include primary terms and secondary terms that are synonyms for the primary terms. From the perspective of the ordering physician, a term's status as primary or secondary is irrelevant. The critical issue is that the ordering physician can guess the name of an orderable correctly. Clinical physicians have to be able to locate the orderable and place that order without delay, confusion, or frustration. In general, the department performing the order (e.g., radiology) can define primary terms according to its internal needs, but the terms must be linked to synonyms that are defined according to the wider, general needs of the hospital and specifically according to the needs of the clinical physician who actually places orders.

Ineffective naming contributes to inefficient patient care and needlessly frustrates physicians using the system. The usual areas that create problems with orderable names are radiology and serology, but the same problem can occur anywhere in a catalog.

The point is not to change the behavior of the radiology department, lab, or pharmacy but to use accepted clinical nomenclature rather than jargon so physicians can place orders easily, quickly, and safely. To put it bluntly, using the correct names for orderables will save time and may save lives.

Simple Rules for Naming Orderables

1. Synonyms must be intuitive and in common use by **clinical** physicians.
2. If a new physician can't find an orderable after three guesses, the orderable name is inappropriate.

POLICY ISSUES

In addition to the problems posed by naming conventions, other complications arise in defining orderables and constructing a usable catalog, many of which have implications for hospital policy and resources. Areas of concern include the efficient use of resources in creating the orderables and the catalog, multiple catalogs and mixed vendors, formal versus informal protocol orders, order entry format requirements, and a host of other predictable issues.

Project Cost Versus Ongoing Clinical Costs

The rationale for defining synonyms is evident, but doing so requires time and effort. Many hospitals have therefore simply left their catalog as it is and ignored the need for clinical synonyms. They do so not because they don't see the value but because they see the cost. Nonetheless, if the project does not bother to spend resources on defining appropriate synonyms, the clinical staff will be forced to spend an inappropriate amount of time searching the system. Not spending the resources initially is a classic case of cost shifting, and the outcome is an inefficient hospital. This same issue pertains to paring down the list of routes, frequencies, doses, and units associated with each orderable. While the system vendor sometimes does so prior to installation, often the onus is on the hospital. This task may involve considerable effort on the part of a hospital's pharmacists and too often is simply ignored. Again, the outcome is an inefficient hospital: If no time is spent up front weeding out options within each orderable, physicians spend countless collective hours doing so every day in every order.

Consider an example. Mylanta is typically given orally (or by gastric tube), yet in one hospital in Iowa, the list of potential routes also includes intravenous and 43 other inappropriate options. Physicians waste clinical time looking for the only appropriate option (they need to scroll through three screens to locate the right

> ### Examples of Inappropriate Orderable Options
> ### (from actual hospital catalogs)
>
> | Orderable | Inappropriate Options |
> |---|---|
> | Mylanta | *Route:* intravenous, rectal, subcutaneous |
> | Insulin | *Units:* centimeters, grams, milligrams, ounces, tabs |
> | Stool culture | *Source:* bilateral tympani, pulmonary artery |
> | Serum helicobacter | *Source:* urine, stool, sputum, abscess, central line |
> | Ancef | *Frequency:* once per week, every 15 minutes |

option in this case), and inclusion of inappropriate routes raises the marginal patient risk that someone might actually attempt to give Mylanta by vein or other incorrect ways. Paring down the list of optional routes removes this risk.

The same logic applies to optional frequencies, doses, and units for each medication. Inappropriate laboratory orderables likewise need to be weeded out, as do radiology orders. The shorter the list of (appropriate) options, the easier it is to place the order, the faster the clinical workflow, and the lower the patient risk.

And yet, the same question of resources applies: Cleanup requires project resources, but if not done, the outcome will be extensive continuing costs to clinical time. In essence, not weeding out orderable options during implementation is an "unfunded mandate" on clinical time.

MULTIPLE CATALOGS

While some hospitals operate nicely with a single catalog, a number of situations force the creation of more complicated catalogs.

The most obvious is that of a multiple-hospital system in which not all of the hospitals have access to the same orderables. While hospital A does toxicology screens in its own lab, hospital B sends its toxicology screens to an outside hospital (or to hospital A). While hospital A has access to a cardiac cath lab (and hence can order an angiography test), hospital B has no such resource and must transfer such patients or forego the exam. Hospitals A and B cannot simply share a catalog without making some adaptations. In such cases, "virtualized" orderables are used. Virtualized order-ables can be seen (and ordered) by a physician at hospital A but cannot be seen (or ordered) by a physician at hospital B.

Similar issues pertain to inpatient pharmacy orderables (lim-ited to the hospital formulary) versus outpatient prescriptions (limited only by what neighborhood pharmacies have in their for-mularies). While some drugs are found only in the inpatient formulary, many nongeneric options are generally available in the outpatient formulary, and this difference must (and can) be accounted for. This same sort of issue (with a slightly different solution) pertains to durable medical equipment orderables, such as home oxygen, wheelchairs, and ostomy supplies.

Finally, some hospitals not only have multiple catalogs forced on them due to having separate vendors for their radiology, phar-macy, and laboratory systems but therefore also must find a way to translate such orders from the normal "up-front" catalog in which the clinical physicians place their orders to the "back-end" catalog of the other system used in radiology, the pharmacy, the labora-tory, and so forth.

Protocols and Informal Orders

Most hospitals have always used (and many continue to use) pro-tocols in normal clinical care. Protocols generally promote efficient patient care by permitting the legal performance of routine and accepted care, although even then they are generally backed up by written (or electronic) protocols that have been vetted by the nursing and/or medical staff. Some of these protocols are unwritten, "informal" orders.

An example of the most informal of such orders is the typical understanding among ED nurses that all patients are assumed to be NPO. In reality, many patients override this understanding by bringing in their own food, but the NPO status is still informally assumed, particularly in cases of abdominal pain, trauma, and so on. During the transition to the electronic world, some hospitals actually incorporate formal orders for such patients to be assigned NPO status, while others leave the informal protocol in place. The same occurs with the informal assumption that all ED patients should have their vital signs checked, independent of any formal order from the ED physician. While this assumption may be backed up by a formal ED protocol, written or otherwise, this is not always the case.

Informal orders are becoming fewer and fewer, but they still exist and—within limits—may be appropriate. Only two questions pertain to the use of informal orders: Do they conform to standards of good patient care, and do they fit within current regulatory requirements?

Protocol orders are of two distinct types: those that must be signed by a licensed physician (signed protocols) and those that don't need to be signed (unsigned protocols). The latter are formally defined protocols that have been adopted by the hospital and fit within the nursing scope of practice, such as administering certain immunizations and routine patient care. Such protocols may be instituted without a physician's signature. Most protocols, however, do require a licensed physician's signature. Examples include the triage protocols used in most EDs and the protocols for managing insulin, alcohol withdrawal, and IV pressor agents. A common issue occurs when the distinction between signed and unsigned protocols is unclear (or not made at all) and the nurse—placing a verbal order from a physician—chooses to enter it as a "protocol order," regardless of which **type** of protocol it is. Terminology varies: One hospital may call all orders requiring a physician's signature *protocols* and call all orders that do not require a physician's signature *standing orders*. The terminology is unimportant as long as it is clear to those using it. My protocol may be your standing order, but trouble ensues unless we are both aware of what we mean.

A related issue is billing for such orders. For example, does the hospital bill for point-of-care tests, and do such tests therefore require a formal physician order? The answer to this question varies from hospital to hospital (and clinic to clinic) and must be discussed and clarified in advance, if only to prevent billing losses. In addition, outpatient orders (and, increasingly, inpatient orders) need to be linked to a diagnosis to be billable.

Order Entry Fields

Every orderable comprises details that clarify it and ensure it is accurately completed. These order entry fields (OEFs) include not only the items described earlier (e.g., route, frequency, dose, source) but also additional details that may not need to be included but frequently are included nonetheless. These unnecessary details slow physician care.

Consider, for example, ordering a chest X-ray. The reason for exam (RFE) is not only reasonable in that it is required by The Joint Commission and needed for billing; it has a clear medical rationale as well: The RFE tells radiologists what they need to look for. A chest X-ray taken because of trauma requires a different evaluation than that required for an X-ray taken because of possible metastases. What about the question of possible patient pregnancy, the use of oxygen, and the method of transport, however? Here, the issue is somewhat different than that of the RFE. In the case of the RFE, the concern may not be present in the chart but only in the mind of the ordering physician who is voicing a clinical suspicion. Details on pregnancy, oxygen, and transport, however, are easily gathered from the chart or other sources and are not resident solely in the mind of the ordering physician. In short, these OEFs are usually—and appropriately and more efficiently—addressed by other means than requiring the ordering physician to fill them out each time.

The general rule is to avoid requiring the ordering physicians to fill in necessary missing details and thus slowing them down when those details can be obtained elsewhere. To put it in terms of patient risk, if the pregnancy status is known (or even if unknown), that information (or lack thereof) resides in the chart. To require the physician to reenter such information not only forces double entry of data but also could cause inconsistent information and errors to be documented. If the patient **is** pregnant, the radiology tech needs to access the chart and act accordingly. Otherwise, the ordering physician could mistakenly fill the OEF with false information (i.e., the patient is not pregnant), and the radiology department might rely on such information rather than on the original data (a positive pregnancy test). The "source of truth" should be the chart, not a secondary interpretation made by an ordering physician. Likewise, details of oxygen use and transport mode are best gathered by looking at the actual oxygen supplied and evaluating the patient directly.

Often the justification for missing required details is that "we've always required that information." This fact does not justify the requirement that the **physician** supply such information when placing the order. For example, coagulation test orders may ask for details (e.g., Is this a baseline value? Is the patient on an anticoagulant?) necessary for clinical evaluation (by the physician) but not necessary to run the test itself (by the laboratory technician). For the former, such details are better accessed via the patient's electronic chart.

Rules of Required OEFs

1. Whenever possible, OEFs should not be empty or missing required details.
2. Avoid entering information that is already documented in the patient's chart or that can be efficiently found elsewhere.

SPECIAL ISSUES

A number of other considerations surface in almost all hospitals when they first move their catalog into the world of CPOE. Diet orders are notoriously hard to define in such a way that they are both flexible and easy to use. How easy is it, for example, for the physician to place an "NPO past midnight" order when the patient is on a regular diet? Does the physician have to cancel the original order? Does the change require a separate communication order? What happens when the patient returns from surgery? Or, in the extreme case, how easy is it to order a diet that is low fat, renal, vegetarian, and for an Orthodox Jew? These and similar issues make it difficult to come up with logical, facile, and intuitive ways of ordering diets and require a surprising amount of thought for such a limited set of orders within the broader catalog.

New drugs are always being developed, and a physician might need to place a pharmacy order that is missing from or not yet included in the catalog. Most hospitals include nonspecific orderables to allow for this possibility, including NF (non-formulary), TNF (template non-formulary), and Misc (miscellaneous) orders.

Another common issue occurs at discharge. Many current systems assume that a patient is an inpatient and then is discharged from medical care. The reality is that many patients are transferred to other hospitals, rehab facilities, or skilled nursing facilities. When discharging patients, physicians generally write prescriptions, but they do not do so when a patient is, for example, going to a nursing home. Physicians indicate which medications (and doses, frequencies, routes, and so on) they think are appropriate, but they do not want to write extended prescriptions and thereby assume both medical and legal responsibility. A physician might, for example, indicate that a patient should probably be continued on oral Flagyl but that this suggestion is only a recommendation and actual therapy is of course up to the receiving physician. Most vendors are now aware of—and trying to solve—this practical problem.

MEDICAL ISSUES

Computerized catalogs and orderables raise several questions that previously were irrelevant or not applicable. Most modern hospitals now use dose range checking (which forbids or warns against physician attempts to order a medication outside the normal range, such as one gram of digoxin) and dosing calculators. The latter are becoming routinely used in pediatric care and for those with limited excretion or metabolism of specific medications. Although many of these calculators are weight based, others are based on body surface area, lean body weight (or dosing weight), or several such factors in combination. Whether implementing or optimizing, hospitals are currently faced with several questions: Which drugs should have built-in dose range checking or dosing calculators? Which units (e.g., dosing weight, actual weight, estimated weight, lean body weight, admission weight) should trigger or be part of dosing calculations? Should rounding rules be automatic? Should such rules be preemptive (i.e., required or advisory)?

In the case of interaction checking, similar questions arise. Most hospitals now limit the types of interactions that trigger alerts to the most severe kinds rather than have all possible interactions trigger alerts to ordering physicians. Many hospitals even are electing to remove specific interactions, such as the alert that fires if a patient is given ketorolac in the ED and then discharged on another oral NSAID, such as ibuprofen. Such an alert is unnecessary and inappropriate because this prescribing behavior is likely to be indicated and expected of good clinical care. When this sort of inappropriate alerting takes place, it not only slows care but also undermines all future alerts: The physician comes to ignore them. Knowing that all previous alerts were apparently irrelevant to decision making, they infer that future alerts will be likewise irrelevant. This normal human inference notwithstanding, some interactions are critical, and we cannot afford to discount all future alerts by permitting random inappropriate alerts to dilute their importance. As with all alerts, the definition of an appropriate alert (interaction checking or otherwise) is one that alters medical care. As discussed in the final chapter of this book, *appropriate alert* should be defined concretely and practically: Not only do we weed out our alerts a priori using logic; we also circle back and weed them out a posteriori on the basis of audits indicating which alerts actually **do** alter care. If an alert never changes medical care, why have it at all?

Duplicate checking is another issue that is more complex than it first appears. Hospitals cannot afford to needlessly waste resources on unnecessary tests, but *unnecessary*—and what constitutes a duplicate order—is difficult to define. There is almost never a medical indication for ordering several identical stool cultures in the same day (a duplicate alert would be appropriate in this case) or for ordering two CBCs five minutes apart (as occurs when an intern and resident both place similar orders), but what about two CBCs placed one day apart? And if the patient is actively bleeding, how close together can such CBCs be placed and still be appropriate rather than unnecessary duplicate orders? Blood cultures are routinely ordered in pairs, making the second blood culture not a duplicate but a standard of care. How then do we define duplicate blood culture orders? Naively, we might suggest that two EKGs ordered five minutes apart are duplicates, but if one minute after the first EKG the patient suddenly develops severe substernal pain, the second EKG is indicated. The upshot is that most duplicate orders are defined on a case-by-case basis and depend on the policy of the hospital.

Many orderables are meant to trigger multiple tasks. When a physician orders nebulized albuterol, the order normally triggers a task for the respiratory therapist (i.e., provide the treatment) and a task for the pharmacist (i.e., supply the albuterol). Such orders are, in general, poorly handled by many vendors and may require some thought on the part of the hospital, particularly orders to the blood bank: While the physician thinks of "give two units of packed red blood cells" as a single order, it may actually encompass several orders (usually at least two, but up to seven at one hospital), including (1) order the type and cross, (2) bring the units to the ward,

(3) ensure an IV access, (4) start saline, (5) obtain patient consent, (6) give the packed red cells, and (7) treat any complications. Any orders that normally trigger multiple tasks must be considered and planned for ahead of time.

The same general principle (i.e., orders are different when they are computerized) applies to "if-then" orders that were normal in the paper world but again require forethought and planning in the computer world. For example, an if-then order might be, "Get a CBC now and check the results. If the hemoglobin is below ten, then order a reticulocyte count in the morning." Again, this type of order is not yet native to CPOE and requires forethought.

KEY POINTS

- Each hospital has its own catalog and orderables. The catalog must be cleaned up and orderables must be defined early in the project and on schedule.
- All orderables must have common, intuitive names (or synonyms) as judged by the **ordering** physician and as reflected in general medical usage.
- Orderables should never have unnecessary OEFs or be missing required details that are easily gathered. Those that do have unnecessary OEFs or are missing required details slow patient care and may increase risk if they require duplicate data entry.
- Orderables' OEFs (e.g., dose, route, frequency, source) must be weeded out to include only appropriate options. This task requires work to be done up front, but it saves far more physician work and speeds patient care while decreasing patient risk.

PART II

Practical Issues

CHAPTER 5

Order Sets, Orders, and Ordering

There is nothing so useless as doing efficiently
that which should not be done at all.

—*Peter Drucker*

DEFINITIONS

Order sets are collections of orders that can be requested as a unit.
For example, an order set called "admission for myocardial infarction" might include orders for admission, diet, nursing care, oxygen, monitoring, routine and stat labs, radiology workup, drugs,
and various consults. Order sets eliminate the need to search for
each component order. In addition, the orders in most order sets
already include default details and do not require the provider to
fill in additional information; in the case of the "admission for
myocardial infarction" order set, for example, the reason for exam
(RFE) included in the component chest X-ray order already would
be set to "myocardial infarction." Different vendors, different IT
departments, and different hospitals use slightly different terms
when referring to order sets, such as *care set*. Some newer types of
order sets have additional functionality and specific names, such as
"PowerPlan" (in the case of Cerner).

Favorite folders are collections of orders that have been saved
by an individual user in a personal file so they can be quickly
retrieved in the future. A nephrologist might, for example, have

a favorite folder that includes laboratory orders for potassium, creatinine, and BUN along with specific dialysates and other orders that are the daily province of nephrology. A cardiologist's favorite folder would likely include orders for EKGs, cardiac enzymes, stress echoes, and others common to cardiology. Favorite folders are idiosyncratic and reflect the way individuals—not departments or hospitals—practice and organize their workflows. I might put an order for abdominal ultrasound in a folder called "radiology," while you might put the same order under the complaint that prompts the order (abdominal pain).

Home folders reflect a department or specialty. They include orders (and order sets) that a specialty or department most commonly use. For an orthopedics department, the home folder would include several useful order sets (e.g., total hip replacement), multiple radiologic procedures (e.g., pre- and post-surgical joint views), relatively few labs, a few antibiotics, and extensive medications for pain (e.g., morphine patient-controlled analgesia [PCA]). In contrast, the home folder for a department of infectious disease would include different order sets (e.g., septic workup), specialty-specific radiology tests (e.g., chest X-ray to rule out pneumonia, ultrasound to rule out abscess), specialty-specific labs to identify organisms (e.g., cultures of blood, urine, and cerebrospinal fluid), and a wide variety of antibiotic, antifungal, and antiviral agents but fewer pain medications than would appear in the home folder of the orthopedics department.

THE RATIONALE FOR ORDER SETS

Orders should be placed efficiently.

From the standpoint of the physician—as opposed to that of the nurse or secretary who **takes** orders—there is nothing as efficient as a simple verbal order. Even from the physician's standpoint, however, there are limits to verbal orders. When physicians are placing dozens of orders, they are less likely to become confused if they can see and organize those orders as they are placed, even in the paper world. Moreover, the risk of misunderstood, illegible, and inadvertent orders climbs with the number of orders placed, as is the case with most admission orders, in which numerous otherwise unrelated orders are placed in a defined sequence. In contradistinction to the physician's preference for the simplicity of the verbal order and individual efficiency, these critical considerations derive from the need to provide safe patient care, adhere to regulatory requirements, and ensure the efficiency of the hospital as a whole.

Given the multiple benefits of placing orders via computer, there is still the issue of how we can maximize physicians' efficiency in placing those orders. To access websites we commonly visit (e.g., Amazon, Google, LinkedIn, Facebook), few of us go through the trouble of typing out the entire web address (e.g., http://www.amazon.com); rather, we click on a single icon or select the URL from a drop-down. The workflow savings are enormous: We accomplish in a click or two what might otherwise require dozens of clicks, and the time we save is likewise enormous. Placing medical orders is precisely the same: **The most efficient way to place an order is by a single click.** The same is true for individual orders and for order sets.

The most inefficient way to place orders is to type the entire name of the order in a search window, click, and then choose additional order details.

If we need to modify an order in an order set, it is more efficient to pull up the order set, select the order, and modify it than to type the name of the order, locate it, and then fill in the missing details.

STANDARDIZATION

Order sets are meant to increase efficiency and shape medical decision making to bring it closer to accepted medical protocols.

Hopefully such protocols are based on objective evidence and are not merely a reiteration of "what we always did in the past." A well-constructed order set is therefore a short compilation of standard orders that speak directly to a specific patient, are based on objective evidence, and are kept up to date. An order set is efficient if a physician can use it in daily clinical practice **with few to no alterations**. In the paper world, written protocols spoke to much the same need and likewise accomplished the dual goal of efficiency and (appropriate) standardization.

Order sets should never attempt to prohibit or absolutely restrict medical care. Patients vary and medicine (one hopes) advances over time. If order sets were to lock in the medical care that was considered appropriate a century ago, we would not be able to order antibiotics, CT scans, or current surgical procedures. Order sets must not only reflect what we currently accept but also be kept current with advances and changes in medical care. We can try to avoid known errors and risks, but we cannot afford to restrict change.

Most modern order sets therefore shape medical treatment by making nonstandard or uncommon orders harder to place than standard and common orders. Realistically, such order sets reflect several inputs. The most obvious input is current physician practice in a hospital. The usual starting point for creating any computerized order set is, therefore, to take the existing paper order set and simply translate it into a similar (though rarely identical) computer order set. Several other inputs also play a role, including regulatory compliance (e.g., with Joint Commission meaningful-use requirements), hospital costs (e.g., based on choice of drugs, equipment, available tests, or procedures), and the current medical literature (i.e., evidence-based medicine).

A specialty's standards cannot be set by other departments. The design of an order set should reflect input from multiple departments and perspectives but must ultimately reflect the standard of care as determined by the physician specialty using that order set. A medical specialty is ethically and medically responsible for defining its own standards of medical care on the basis of accepted norms and cannot abrogate that responsibility to other departments.

As an example, while both cardiologists and pharmacists might appropriately offer input on an ED order set—such as an order set dealing with the care of patients with acute myocardial infarction—the ultimate responsibility for the appropriateness of emergency care lies with the current evidence-based practices of emergency medicine as reflected in a national or global consensus of that specialty. Cardiologists can no more determine the appropriate standards of emergency medicine than emergency physicians can determine the appropriate standards of cardiology; the key is respect for one another's expertise. It is appropriate for areas of specialty to seek and offer input, but it is not appropriate for one specialty to dictate unilaterally to another. Likewise, while endocrinologists should offer guidance on how a hospitalist order set addresses insulin usage, responsibility for that order set remains that of the hospitalists. In the same sense, respiratory therapy, anesthesia, infectious disease, and other inputs are to be sought and valued, but each specialty must have and must accept responsibility for its own order sets and for the standards of care reflected in those sets.

Finally, as noted in Chapter 4, not all paper-based orders can be translated directly into computer-based order sets. **Computer order sets are almost never exact translations of paper order sets.** The two most common exceptions to easy translation are dual-tasking orders (e.g., nebulized albuterol is an order that tasks both the respiratory and the pharmacy departments; blood bank orders frequently comprise three to seven different orders to administer a single blood product) and if-then orders (e.g., if hemoglobin is below ten, a reticulocyte count is ordered; the results of the first order determine whether to place a second order).

Computerized order sets are different from paper order sets in several ways. We can link order sets to hospital protocols or to active websites; we can include subsets of orders, which can be ordered within the original order set; and we can add drop-downs with multiple options (e.g., drug doses). We can include pre-checked defaults but also permit physicians to uncheck any item they don't want to order, we can provide alerts based on rules, and we can save personal versions of basic order sets. In short, computer order sets offer additional features and flexibility not present in paper versions of what might otherwise be the "same" order set.

Nomenclature

Although at first sight the issue of naming conventions may seem trivial, it is exactly the sort of detail that determines whether providers will actually **use** the order sets. Experience shows that providers use order sets that they can easily find and ignore order sets whose names make them difficult to find. The absolute rule of thumb is simple: **Order set names must be intuitive and consistent.**

Order sets should be named according to most of the same criteria for naming orderables: Names should be intuitive, and the naming rules should be consistent. In both cases—the need to be (1) intuitive and (2) consistent—the rationale is the same. The goal is efficiency and ease of use. We need to ensure that any physician—whether newly hired, consulting on an unfamiliar ward, rushing to surgery, or tired after a long night shift—can instantly find an order set without clicking, searching, or asking someone, and certainly without frustration or confusion. Order sets should be named in such a way that physicians find exactly what they are looking for on their first attempt.

Rules of Naming Order Sets

1. Order sets should be named in such a way that the user's first guess is the right guess.
2. The naming convention should be consistent across all order sets.

In many hospitals, this rule is not followed, and the results can be both frustrating and occasionally funny, but poorly chosen names are still inexcusable. They slow down care and increase the risk of inappropriate ordering.

Avoid jargon and idiosyncratic technicalities. Avoid abbreviations—particularly idiosyncratic abbreviations—or naming conventions that are unfamiliar to those who will actually place the orders. They may be obvious to the person naming order sets in a warm, dry committee room but may not be obvious to the harried, tired, worried physician who, at 2 a.m., is attempting to find an order set to treat his pediatric trauma patient. The name must be intuitively obvious **to the clinician using the order set**. Once again, clinical input is essential, and the outcome must be intuitive and consistent. Clinical predictability is the key.

Consistency is needed not for its own sake but rather to permit rapid and accurate use by clinicians who are not used to a particular order set. If a surgeon accustomed to using surgical order sets is admitting a pediatric patient and is faced with an unfamiliar pediatric order set, the name of that order set should reflect its content to the surgeon and to any other physician who is considering using it.

Misleading Order Set Titles

In one small community hospital, there was an order set named "ED Abd Pn Acute Fe." One physician interpreted this name as "acute iron (Fe) ingestion." The actual meaning was "emergency department abdominal pain acute female," and the corresponding male version of this order set was named "ED Abd Pn Acute Male." While acute iron ingestion does cause abdominal pain, the inappropriate use of the idiosyncratic abbreviation "Fe" for female was unnecessary, as well as misleading. In both cases, the abbreviation "Pn" for pain also was both unnecessary and potentially confusing.

> ### Examples of Typical Nomenclature Patterns for Order Sets
>
> - *Pattern:* [Condition] [Disposition] [Location]
>   —*Example:* CHF Admission ICU
> - *Pattern:* [Department] [Procedure] [Pre/Post] [Disposition]
>   —*Example:* ORTHO Hip Replacement Pre-Op Admission

In most hospitals, the nomenclature is well defined, standardized, and eminently understandable. Most order sets begin with a short, common abbreviation that reflects the department or specialty, such as ED, SURG, PEDS, ICU, or ORTHO. This abbreviation is followed by a sequence of terms reflecting the use of the order set for admission, transfer, pre-op or post-op patients, diagnosis or complaint, and so on. The acid test of the value of a nomenclature should be: If we ask any staff physician to guess what the order set is used for, will he or she guess correctly? If the answer is yes, the order sets are well named; if no, it's time to go back and start over.

Internal Organization of Order Sets

Order sets require not only a standard nomenclature but a standard internal organization as well. Generally, this organization reflects a hospital's historical precedent. The pattern by which the orders are organized derives from the paper-based precedent. One example of an organization pattern might be: admission, diagnosis, condition, vital signs, activity, nursing, diet, IVs, medications, labs, and so on.

Any of various common patterns can be used, such as those derived or adapted from the *Washington Manual*; from Zynx Health, ProVation Medical, or BMJ Group; or from any other common framework. In general, the organization of the order set

> **Examples of Order Sets from Various Hospitals**
>
> ED Abdominal Pain, Female
>
> ED Toxicology Workup
>
> ED Chest Pain
>
> ED Common Labs
>
> ED Plain Films
>
> SURG Post-operative Hip Replacement
>
> ANES PACU Orders
>
> HOSP Septic Workup
>
> HOSP ICU Admission
>
> HOSP CHF Therapy
>
> MED General Medical Admission
>
> MED Common Antibiotics
>
> PEDS Febrile Child
>
> PEDS Seizure Workup
>
> PEDS Admission
>
> OB—Normal Vag Delivery

should be similar (or even precisely the same) as that previously used in the hospital (to avoid confusion and unnecessary change), but in many cases the organization might be altered for at least two logical considerations:

1. The hospital may have a commercial subscription to a source of order sets (such as its software vendor or other evidence-based source), in which case the organization of the order sets might reasonably be that used by the commercial source.
2. The hospital may feel that its historical pattern was ineffective or unsafe and should be updated or changed to improve medical care.

To address the latter consideration—efficacy or safety—the hospital might decide to place medication orders toward the top of the order set to minimize the risk of inadvertently placed medication orders (an "error of commission"). Providers may order medications inadvertently if they don't scroll all the way down to see the pre-checked medication orders. In some hospitals, this risk has also been addressed by a policy of not permitting pre-checked medication orders at all, although this policy undercuts the purpose of using order sets (i.e., to shape medical therapy into optimal, evidence-based care), slows medical care, and increases the risk of inadvertent omission of necessary patient medications (an "error of omission").

Prohibition of pre-checked medication orders is an example of a narrow focus on risk to the detriment of workflow and all other considerations of effective patient care (such as the quality and timeliness of that care). As ever, naïve considerations of risk can inadvertently increase patient risk.

While many hospitals still construct their own order sets from scratch or from their existing, internal order sets, the majority of hospitals now use order sets from one of three outside sources: EHR vendors (e.g., Cerner, Epic), order set vendors (e.g., Zynx), or other hospitals that share their order sets. Many vendors now offer "starter" order sets. In some cases, these sets have been constructed by the vendor, while in other cases they represent a continuously increasing library of order sets shared by all of the vendor's clients. In the latter case, hospitals may be encouraged to use the vendor's library of order sets in exchange for entering their own order sets into the vendor's library for future use by other clients. Vendor libraries ensure a ready source of order sets that have actually been in clinical use (with some implication for potential clinical quality in that previous clinical use at other hospitals may already have identified and corrected any medical errors).

Examples of Order Set Categories (simplified and adapted)

Zynx categories:
- Condition
- Vital signs
- Activity
- Nursing orders
- Patient education
- Respiratory
- Diet
- IV
- Medications
- Blood
- Laboratory
- Diagnostic imaging
- Consults

Washington Manual categories:
- Admitting
- Diagnosis
- Condition
- Vital signs
- Activity
- Nursing orders
- Diet
- Allergies
- Laboratory
- IV
- Sedatives
- Medications

For creating (and maintaining) order sets, many EHR vendors also offer a formal framework in which to review, edit, and achieve consensus among multiple inputs, as do most order set vendors. Zynx, for example, has an "AuthorSpace" in which an order set can be designed and built—complete with orderables, order sentences, pre-checks, and so forth—and then reviewed by other parties (e.g., pharmacists, nurses, specialty physicians). While one author may "own" the order set as it is in progress, others can access the order set to add comments and offer suggestions for improvement. Order sets can be built using any number of formats, including paper and Excel spreadsheets, but it is far more common and easier to build and track order sets that are created in a formal computer framework intended for such use.

Commercially available sources of order sets offer two additional benefits not usually found in order sets offered by EHR software vendors. These subscription order sets are

1. **updated** regularly to reflect best practices, and
2. **linked** to current literature reflecting those best practices.

Horror Story on Having Order Sets Only for Some Departments

A client decided to make order set development optional for its medical staff and to address need as it arose post-conversion. At the time of conversion, the ED had developed order sets for its major needs, but only two non-ED order sets had been created. Two years later, the ED was at 95 percent CPOE and the entire medical staff (counting the ED physicians) was at 6 percent. In an effort to improve the medical staff's numbers, hospital administration is pressuring the ED physicians to increase their use of CPOE while the rest of the medical staff is merely being encouraged to use CPOE.

In Zynx's order sets, for example, orderables can incorporate icons (blue ribbons) that link to national performance measures or to Zynx's own evidence summaries. The linkage to current medical literature is especially useful to academic institutions, where the training of residents and students provides an impetus to have such references available concomitantly with delivering patient care. Finally, many commercial order set vendors do not map one-to-one to EHR vendor order sets. Zynx, for example, does not currently offer multiphase order set design, a feature that is useful in the PowerPlan in Cerner's EHR. This observation can be generalized: Most commercially available order sets require some effort and "translation" to be used in EHRs.

RESOURCES NEEDED TO DESIGN ORDER SETS

The single largest headache—and the largest time consumer—of any EHR implementation is the creation of order sets. Almost inevitably, at least at the onset of the project, there is incredulity that creating order sets can consume so many person-hours. The best estimate is that—if starting from scratch—the average order set takes around 80 person-hours to finish. How can creation of an order set possibly take so much time and, therefore, money? There are two major sources of work:

1. Obtaining design input from disparate viewpoints
2. Obtaining political consensus on the final design

Design input comes not merely from physicians but also from other hospital personnel; political consensus comes not merely from the order set committee but also from the medical executive committee, the pharmacy and therapeutics committee, and other standing political groups. Yet despite the fact that order set design is resource intensive, the clinical utility of order sets makes them cost-effective as well as necessary to good patient care.

The typical hospital—at the time of initial implementation—has several dozen order sets (e.g., 50 to 75) in the ED and a few hundred order sets (e.g., 200 to 300) for inpatient care throughout the hospital (exclusive of the ED but covering all other inpatient specialties). While some of these order sets will be discontinued over time (see the section on maintenance later in the chapter), the overall trend is to increase the number of order sets, particularly during the initial year or two post-implementation.

The design of an order set not only reflects its medical service (e.g., surgery, cardiology, emergency, gynecology) but also requires input from pharmacy, nursing, dietary, respiratory, EKG, radiology, blood bank, laboratory, regulatory, registration, and quality assurance personnel. Having all these groups in every meeting of an order set subcommittee is not only impossible but also extremely wasteful of resources. Likewise, the political vetting of order sets cannot be delayed until "the next meeting of the medical executive committee two months from now." Moreover, order sets must be carefully matched to the orderables catalog and edited to fit into the computer world. This task usually requires that either the vendor or the IT department be kept in the loop, another potential cause of delay.

Inherent in the limits of deadlines (and budgets) is the knowledge that we cannot build an infinite number of order sets. Which ones have priority? Priorities are set by hospital billing (e.g., the DRGs most commonly billed for), ease of building (e.g., translating current paper order sets), political considerations (e.g., physicians who admit the most patients), regulatory risks (e.g., the last visit of The Joint Commission), and ease of use (e.g., "convenience" order sets).

THE WELL-DESIGNED ORDER SET

Order sets are designed to be used. They are not meant to be all-inclusive, to force the user to perform an action, or to preclude any potential error of medical judgment. Order sets can shape actions, but they cannot enforce them; they can encourage good medical care, but they cannot mandate it; they can minimize risks, but they cannot eliminate them.

Order sets are not "cookbook medicine," but they do provide useful recipes. A well-designed order set is meant to **shape and suggest**, but it cannot replace medical judgment. Any committee that thinks otherwise—and tries to enforce a **single standard without any possible exception**—is deluding itself and undermining the quality of patient care. A good order set can't force physicians to do the right thing, but it can improve the

---

Which Order Sets Do We Need to Design?

The following steps can help hospitals prioritize the order sets they need to build:

1. Gather current paper order sets and prioritize them for frequency of use and for ease of translation (into a computer version).
2. Create a list of the most common DRGs billed for in the past 12 months (e.g., congestive heart failure, diabetes).
3. Create a list of physicians who admitted the most patients in the past 12 months and the order sets they will apply to the patients they admit.
4. Have quality assurance prioritize current hospital risks on the basis of litigation, Joint Commission requirements, and so on (which order sets would address and mitigate these concerns?).
5. Create a list of order sets that will make providers' jobs easier. Ask the laboratory for a list of the two dozen most commonly ordered labs and likewise ask the pharmacy and radiology for their most common orders.

---

quality of care and make it easier—rather than harder—for the physician to do the right thing.

A well-designed order set is terse, consensual, and backed by clinical data. The best order set represents the best available data on what constitutes excellent care for the majority of patients. The design should be based on current medical literature, common sense, and current clinical practice at the institution. As the literature changes, so should the order set. A pneumonia order set in which antibiotics haven't changed during the past two years is already out of date.

Common sense should reflect reality: While it might seem reasonable to pre-check an order for a chest X-ray in an "admit for community-acquired pneumonia" order set, most patients are admitted for this diagnosis because of the chest X-ray they **already had taken**. The X-ray is the reason they are being admitted to the hospital in the first place.

Actual, current clinical practice also should play a role in the design of order sets. Different hospitals offer different services, have different referral patterns, and serve different patient populations. To expect a single "admit for myocardial infarction" order set to function in all hospitals is unrealistic. One hospital has a cardiac catheterization service, while another does not; one is a small community hospital that transfers all heart patients, whereas another is a large tertiary, university hospital that accepts such transfers. Demographics, finances, commonly treated diseases, and patterns of complications differ among hospitals. Order sets should reflect local reality while striving to improve that reality.

Never include orders that "might be useful." The number of orders in an order set is at least as important as the orders themselves. An ideal order set should be viewable hands-free (i.e., without having to scroll or click). During the design phase, the suggestion that a particular order "might be useful" should prompt suspicion and probably exclusion of the suggested order. Inclusion of orders that might be useful invariably leads to "kitchen sink" order sets that include all possible orders but are unwieldy and unused. Not only does each scroll or click slow down medical care; it also increases the risk that something will be missed (or ordered inadvertently) because it is on a different screen. This issue has been repeatedly leveled at order set vendors, who tend to include all possible orders rather than only the most important orders. On the one hand, this comprehensiveness is one of the advantages of commercial order sets, despite the absence of many orderables (e.g., certain drugs) from most hospital formularies; you know you won't leave anything out. But it also is a weakness; you need to aggressively edit each commercial order set to accord with your own formulary and catalog. Commercial order sets should never be used as is. They must be strenuously edited to reflect realistic clinical use.

The shorter the order set, the better; every scroll or click increases the risk of error. The fewer the screens per order set, the easier (and safer) it is to use. While the **ideal** order set might be fitted into a single screen, most order sets can easily be fitted into two or at most three screens. If an order set is too large to fit into two to three screens, it should be reconsidered and—if possible—shortened or divided into two or more order sets.

The larger the order set, the more time it takes to use and to place orders. The well-designed order set is not only well organized, backed by data, and terse but also pre-checked and defaulted in such a way as to both minimize wasted time and "push" good quality care. For example, an order set for elective intubation might include a pre-checked chest X-ray with the RFE defaulted to "post-intubation X-ray to check tube position." In general, the rule is that if the order usually is (or should be) done, it should be pre-checked; if the order usually isn't (or shouldn't be) done, it shouldn't be pre-checked. Consider the time lost (and the patient risk) if these rules are not followed. If a particular order is not pre-checked but is used in 99 percent of cases, 99 percent of physicians will be forced to waste time checking this order and there is considerable risk that this clinically appropriate item won't be ordered for some patients.

> **The Well-Designed Order Set**
>
> Well-designed order sets have
>
> - no more than three screens,
> - no more than 75 orders (40 in the case of the ED),
> - the most common orders at the top of each category,
> - default order sentences (particularly medication orders), and
> - default order entry fields (OEFs) (every OEF that can be defaulted **is** defaulted).

Rare exceptions are reasonable. While a specific high-risk medication (e.g., heparin) might be ordered for the majority of patients, if that medication is pre-checked (particularly if it is not on the first viewable screen of the order set), there is substantial risk that a patient may be prescribed a medication that is unnecessary or dangerous. Most hospitals pre-check all frequently used orders, including medications, but may still exempt certain high-risk medications. As noted earlier, this approach has its own risks, notably the risk of inadvertent omission and the consequent risk of substandard patient care and patient injury or death.

Caveat: Prohibiting pre-checked medication orders is not the same as preventing risk. In some orders, there may be a default (e.g., an IV saline rate of 125 ml per hour), but the program may also allow additional drop-down options (e.g., a rate of 60, 200, or 1000 ml per hour). This same approach may be used for common diets (e.g., regular diets on medical floors, but NPO in the post-anesthesia care unit), medications (e.g., 800 ibuprofen, with drop-down options for 200, 400, and 600 mg), activities, timing of labs (e.g., stat, qAM), and so forth. Good design mandates that the default be the most common option and that other options (limited to around six) represent realistic patterns of use.

The final important design consideration is inclusion of such defaults, especially when the details of the order are required, such as when the physician is required to insert a reason for ordering a test. Prevention of missing details is part of the definition of a well-designed order set. If a physician orders a single chest X-ray for a patient (outside of an order set), he or she will be required to give an RFE (e.g., chest pain, shortness of breath). This reason won't be the default when a single chest X-ray is ordered because the computer doesn't know why the physician is placing the order. In an order set, on the other hand, such details can often—and should—be included as defaults, even though they cannot be specified in the order when used outside the order set. In an order set titled "Admit for CHF," the chest X-ray is being ordered for a known reason (i.e.,

---

I Wonder Where You Got That Stool Sample

In one national hospital chain, physicians were required to select from an extensive list of possible origins for every stool they ordered for culture. This list included not only stool (the appropriate choice, which, due to its position in the alphabetical order of the long series of drop-down items, appeared several screens after the first) but also urine, blood, bilateral tympanum, and pulmonary artery, among other bizarre options. The task of finding and selecting stool from among such options wasted physician time and delayed patient care, and inclusion of such choices severely undercut the credibility of the system. As one physician put it, "If I can get stool from my patient's pulmonary artery, then sending it for culture isn't going to help my patient very much. And if the designers of this system think that stool comes from the pulmonary artery, why would I ever think I can trust this system to support good medical care?"

to establish the degree of failure or other co-disease), so this reason needs to be the default for the X-ray order in this order set. The same logic applies to most other orders in an order set.

Rule of thumb: *All* **details should be included as defaults unless impossible.** We have seen hospitals in which the physician ordering a complete blood count is required to note that the source is blood (not urine) or that the source of a urinalysis is urine (not blood). Such poorly designed order sets undermine not only the credibility of the system (and the hospital) but also the quality of care by slowing the time it takes to treat patients and increasing the probability of error. There is no excuse for inept order sets.

Bad order set design is bad patient care.

TYPES OF ORDER SETS

Order sets are created for several reasons, and their content reflects their variable uses. The majority of order sets are defined by specialty. Surgical order sets, for example, might include order sets for surgical admission or for the treatment of particular surgical conditions. Such order sets might therefore include "SURG Admit Acute Abdomen," "SURG Pre-Op Cholecystectomy," and "SURG Post-Op Colostomy." In addition, this same principle pertains to order sets aimed at well-defined procedures, such as rapid-sequence intubation, lumbar puncture, and colonoscopy.

Convenience order sets, which are made up of similar types of orders (e.g., common laboratory tests, commonly used antibiotics), enable physicians to easily locate single orders (or a small number of orders). If, for example, a physician wants to find orders for a complete blood count and a basic metabolic panel, it is easier to pull up an order set of common laboratory tests than it is to search through an order set intended for an admission. Similarly, many hospitals construct order sets containing nothing but commonly used antibiotics, often broken down by region of the body, such as central nervous system, soft tissue, pulmonary system, and gastrointestinal system. Likewise, ED and ambulatory physicians often order single plain films of a bone (e.g., three views of the ankle) and, rather than typing out the name of the film and searching for it, can pull up an order set of common X-rays and easily click on the X-ray they need. Orders for plain films often include a default RFE as well. In some cases, a group of orders naturally needs to be lumped together, as in the case of respiratory therapy or blood bank orders. In the latter case, the group might include not only an order for the blood product to be given (e.g., packed red blood cells, fresh frozen plasma, leukocyte-poor or irradiated red cells) but also an order for a type and cross or a type and screen (and the need to "stay ahead" two units), a peripheral access order (e.g., insertion of an IV catheter), an order for the fluid to be used in that access (e.g., saline), an order for patient or family consent, orders addressing potential reactions to the blood product administration (e.g., antihistamines), and an order to actually **give** the blood product to the patient. In one memorable case of a hospital that lacked this final order, several units of blood simply sat at the patient's bedside for six hours solely because—while there were orders to type and cross the blood, deliver it to the ward, and use saline via a large-bore peripheral IV—no one had an order to actually administer the blood. **If well designed, convenience order sets not only are convenient but also save time, prevent frustration, and promote better patient care.**

A number of hospitals have used order sets to address their regulatory concerns, although other approaches (e.g., building required actions into routine order sets, using rules and alerts) are evolving with the rapidly changing regulatory environment. Order sets also have been used to clarify discharge plans, to organize potential dietary choices, and for other specific therapeutic needs, including insulin therapy and anticoagulation.

IV solutions

Laboratory tests

Medications (often grouped by type of medication)

Antibiotics (often grouped by type of infection)

X-rays (especially plain films, often including a default RFE)

Ultrasounds (often specified by clinical indication)

CTs (often specified by clinical indication)

MRIs (often specified by clinical indication)

Pain medications (often including PCAs)

Nursing orders

Procedures (generally non-operating-room-based procedures)

Consultation services

Respiratory care

Blood bank orders

MAINTAINING ORDER SETS

Order sets typically go through a standard cycle: They are designed, tweaked, accepted, entered into the system, and used by clinicians, and then—as time goes by—they are redesigned, updated, and reused. Control of this process requires both a responsible political structure and a set of parameters linked to each order set. On the whole, the number of order sets in a hospital's system increases over time, but some will be discontinued, and all should be reevaluated and improved on the basis of actual care.

The key elements of the political structure are described in Chapter 3. In essence, it consists of not only the order set committee and other associated clinical committees (e.g., medical executive committee, pharmacy and therapeutics committee) but also the executive suite, specialists (e.g., orthopedists, neurologists), and other relevant hospital interests (e.g., nursing, pharmacy, laboratory, radiology, registration). These groups must work in coordination to maintain useful and medically appropriate order sets.

The job of the order set committee is to meld these interests, ensuring that each order set represents not only good patient care in its respective specialty but also the best interests of the hospital as a whole. The committee also ensures that the format is consistent with accepted order set conventions and current EHR function—that is, the order set actually works in clinical practice. Many times, the role of the order set committee consists of enforcing priorities and conventions, as well as convincing specialties to respond in a timely fashion. Hospitals typically have at least one specialty or department that is unresponsive to requests for physician input yet quick to complain when the resulting order sets are not medically appropriate for its use. The fact that the specialty/department was "too busy to provide input" has little effect on the volume of the complaint. Enforcing such input can be politically difficult, contribute to the overall cost of designing and maintaining order sets, and delay implementation.

As occurs in the design phase, so too in the maintenance phase: A common political error is to allow the input of one department to ride roughshod over another department. Pharmacy input is critical, but the pharmacy cannot unilaterally determine the best drug or most effective dose for actual clinical use; both the responsibility and the liability for that decision remain with the specialty that is using—and should therefore be designing and maintaining—that order set. The same error occurs if we permit one department to have jurisdiction over the order sets of another. Input is to be encouraged and respected, but **each specialty defines and is responsible for its standards of medical care**.

Politics notwithstanding, each order set also has specific parameters that must be tracked to maintain medical quality. The most obvious of these parameters is the age of the order set. A typical order set requires reevaluation—and probably revision—every year or so. Some order sets (e.g., "Admit for Pneumonia" or "Common Antibiotics") might best be reviewed every six months, while others (e.g., "Common Labs") might be more conservatively managed. A date of last review should be documented for each order set and, by implication, a due date for reevaluation assigned.

In addition, each order set should have an owner who is usually, but not necessarily, a physician. In the case of an order set such as "Admit for Stroke," the physician owner might be a neurologist. The owner takes part in the review of an order set and—should there be any questions as to why it was designed a certain way—can explain the medical rationale behind the initial design. Moreover, the owner is usually a provider who frequently uses the order set and hence has a strong interest in ensuring that it reflects current best practice and is realistic for local conditions.

Finally, order sets should be evaluated for actual use. Data should be collected not only on how often the order set is used but also on how often the orders **within** the order set are used. If an order set has been used only once during the past 12 months, it probably should be retired from the catalog. If the order set was used hundreds of times initially but almost never recently, it needs to be evaluated to see why it is no longer as useful (did best practice change?). Within the order set, if an order is defaulted as unchecked but data show that physicians are checking it 90 percent of the time, should it be pre-checked? If an order is pre-checked but physicians uncheck it every time they use it, should it be unchecked or even deleted altogether? Likewise, if we discover that every time physicians request order set A, they also order lab test B, shouldn't we include that lab test in that order set? These data—order set usage and the **pattern** of ordering—enable us to tailor order sets for clinical use, thereby reducing physician time and improving patient care.

Order sets are like any other part of medical care: They change over time and should be adapted to current recommendations and actual workflow, with an eye toward improving the quality of patient care.

PERSONAL FAVORITE ORDERS

Most systems permit physicians to keep a personal list of their favorite orders, including common details such as dose, route, rate, and RFE. While order sets can be extremely useful, even convenience order sets cannot fully address the need for onetime orders or fine-tune patient ordering. As a common example, hospitalists generally employ an order set to admit their patients the first day but then use onetime orders (generally kept in a favorite file) to place single laboratory orders thereafter. Most hospitalists go one step further and divide their laboratory orders into different folders: one for onetime lab tests and another for daily lab tests. Their medical workflow defines how they construct and use their favorite order folders, and the same is generally true of all specialists. While this pattern of usage is almost universal, it has little impact on implementation and optimization of a system, with a few caveats:

1. When feasible, have providers construct favorites before conversion.
2. The IT department should never erase favorite folders unless doing so is unavoidable, and then only after communicating with the users.
3. Communicate catalog changes so that users may adapt their favorites.
4. Whenever possible, construct departmental home folders in addition to physicians' favorite folders.

DEPARTMENTAL HOME FOLDERS

While most systems support individual favorite orders, most systems can also support home folders for each specialty or hospital department. Each department has its own typical workflow. Orthopedists tend to order certain radiology tests, a narrow number of common antibiotics, and predictable pain medications. These orders are entirely different from those typical of the hospitalist, emergency physician, or pediatrician. A cardiologist may have a folder of his own favorite orders, but cardiologists—as a group—may also commonly place certain orders, and these typical orders can be built into the system. As a cardiologist, I can set my home folder to that of "cardiology" so that when I go to place an order, I first see items that are typical of my practice, not items I rarely or never order. Inclusion of departmental home folders speeds practice and makes physicians more willing to use the system.

A typical hospital has a dozen or more departmental home folders, depending on its size, the number of physicians in its departments, and the ability of its system to support such folders. Departments that commonly have home folders include surgery (with or without folders for specialties, such as neurosurgery, ophthalmology, and trauma), emergency, ICU (and/or hospitalists), pediatrics, OB/GYN, and internal medicine (with or without folders for specialties, such as cardiology, nephrology, and infectious disease).

Each home folder typically includes subfolders for commonly used order sets, lab tests, medications, radiology orders, and perhaps procedures. The "common labs" subfolder, for example, may well contain several dozen lab orders, while the home folder contains only a mere dozen lab orders that are in daily use. Likewise, the "common meds" subfolder may contain several dozen orders, while the home folder includes a mere dozen meds; the "common radiology orders" subfolder may include dozens of X-ray orders, while the home folder contains a dozen or so of the most used X-ray orders. The point is to put the most common orders (for each specialty) on the default home page so that as soon as physicians go to place an order, they see exactly the orders they are most likely to actually use without having to click through screens. Orders that are less commonly used can be placed in a "less commonly used" subfolder (requiring physicians to click on that folder to access them), while orders that are rarely used can be typed in and searched for (which takes the most time but is done the least often).

Individual orders on the home page (labs, meds, and radiology) are usually separated by visual markers (such as asterisks, lines, or spaces) to make them easy to find. Within these categories, orders are arranged alphabetically for easy retrieval. There is a common temptation to arrange them by frequency of use, which appears reasonable but actually tends to slow physicians down. The problem is that while a physician may look at the top of the list for the lab he orders every day, when he is looking for a urinalysis he is unaware that this order is the 37th most likely order, so he's forced to wade through all the other items while trying to spot "U-R-I-N. . . ." In this case, it is actually far easier to search alphabetically than to search by frequency. There are two exceptions to this recommendation: (1) If there are only half a dozen items, the arrangement is irrelevant because the eye can search them in a single glance, and (2) if physicians have become used to a particular arrangement of items on paper over the years, this same arrangement might reasonably be maintained in the computer world.

Departmental home folders are one of the most effective tools for ensuring physician adoption of an EHR system. These folders are an extension of physicians' favorite folders but different in a few ways. First, individual users do not have to build departmental home folders. While most vendors, IT departments, and trainers stress the importance of saving your favorites, not all physicians do so, even with prompting and one-on-one help. Moreover, those least likely to put in the effort to save their personal favorites are usually those who are having the most difficulty with the system. Departmental home folders are "instant" favorites from the day of conversion and allow even the most technology-averse physician to place routine orders quickly and efficiently. Adoption becomes simple.

Second, departmental home folders—like order sets—permit the hospital or the department to shape physician practice into a presumably well-founded standard and potentially improve the quality (and lower the cost) of medical care. For example, if several antibiotics are available but only one (the most effective, least costly, or both) is present in the departmental home folder and defaults are already set for dose, route, frequency, and all other order details, most physicians will follow the path of least resistance and order the suggested medication at the suggested dose. Efficient, one-click ordering can be used to encourage physicians to order certain tests, medications, or procedures. An obvious analogy is the use of the favorites feature in web browsers. Most of us do not go to the trouble of typing in the complete web addresses, including the prefix http://www, of sites we commonly visit. Rather, we click on icons that take us directly to our favorite news, sports, shopping, and weather sites. The same is true of ordering: There is seldom any reason to fill out routine OEFs for orders we place identically every day. We should be "clicking on the icon"—in this case, selecting the one-click order that immediately comes up in our departmental home folder.

The third difference is that departmental home folders, unlike favorite folders, can be constructed with panels, headers, and other visual aids that enable physicians to rapidly locate and place routine daily orders or order sets. Vendor design simply doesn't support these features for favorite folders.

CAVEAT: CLINICAL LIMITATIONS OF ORDER SETS

There is a tendency to believe that order sets (as opposed to home folders) are the best way to standardize care and establish the most efficient workflow. While this belief is roughly accurate, it overlooks several facts and significant clinical realities.

First, departmental home folders can play a key role in standardizing care (independent of order sets) in that home folders offer standard orders, standard dosages, and standard workups, albeit not as a structured unit, such as an order set. The fact that only a single click is required to order a particular antibiotic and dose goes a long way toward standardizing that antibiotic over another choice that might require typing a full name, searching,

Sample Departmental Home Folders

📁 ED CareSets

📁 ED Common Lab

📁 ED Common Medications

📁 ED Common Radiology

CBC
CPK isoenzymes
Drug screen, urine
Troponin
Urinalysis
Etc.
Etc.
Etc.

POWERPLANS

▶ ED Abdominal Pain

▶ ED Chest Pain

▶ ED Dyspnea

▶ ED OB/GYN

▶ ED Pediatrics

▶ ED Trauma

MEDICATIONS

Acetaminophen
Albuterol
Amoxicillin
Ancef
Aspirin
Azithromycin
Etc.
Etc.
Etc.

LABORATORIES

Acetaminophen level
Amylase
BMP
CMP

RADIOLOGY

☐ CT Abdomen w/ + w/o Contrast
CT Chest w/ + w/o Contrast
CT Head or Brain w/ + w/o Contrast
☐ CT Pelvis w/ + w/o Contrast
MRI Abdomen w/ + w/o Contrast
☐ MRI Brain w/ + w/o Contrast
MRI Chest w/ + w/o Contrast
☐ US Abdomen Complete
☐ US Pelvis Non-OB Complete
US Pregnancy Limited
XR Abdomen AP
XR Abdomen Series w/Chest 1 View
XR Ankle Complete Left
XR Ankle Complete Right
XR Chest 1 View
    T;N,Stat,Portable,Once
☐ XR Chest 2 Views
    T;N,Stat,Portable,Once
XR Forearm 2 Views Left
XR Forearm 2 Views Right
XR Skull Complete
XR Spine Cervical 2 or 3 Views
XR Wrist Complete Left
XR Wrist Complete Right

clicking on drop-downs, and filling in several OEFs. Departmental home folders significantly shape ordering behavior.

Second, much of medical care is not amenable to the order set paradigm. The most common use for order sets is for defined procedures, admissions, and well-structured workups. Order sets are less common, less effective, and less efficient for unstructured workups (as is often the case for certain emergency patients) or for "one-off" orders (as is typical of hospital care one to two days after admission or one to two days after surgery).

In short, order sets are appropriate and useful and may even be considered a prime requisite for effective CPOE, but they have limitations and should not be considered the only or even the single most effective way of delivering care, even standardized care. Order sets are a key feature of good medical care, but their use does not—per se—define quality medical care. Optimal use of an EHR includes the use of order sets but also must include efficient access to departmental and personal favorite orders to ensure physicians can hone medical care to best serve their patients.

KEY POINTS

- Order sets must have an
  —intuitive and consistent nomenclature, and
  —intuitive and consistent internal organization.
- Order sets are well designed and useful if they contain
  —the minimum number of orders consistent with daily use, and
  —pre-checked orders with defaulted OEFs whenever feasible.
- Considerable effort is required to build and maintain order sets.
- Departmental home folders are key to easy adoption and efficient ordering.

CHAPTER 6

Workflow and Changing Behaviors

In a chronically leaking boat, energy devoted to
changing vessels is more productive
than energy devoted to patching leaks.

—*Warren Buffett*

FROM THE CLINICAL perspective, implementation comprises
two major tasks: constructing order sets and understanding workflow. Constructing order sets may be more time intensive, but
understanding workflow is more critical to success. A hospital could
go live without order sets—feasible, but not recommended—but
a hospital that tries to go live without giving any thought to the
changing workflow is about to go headlong over a high cliff. The
object of studying workflows is to identify all of the "potholes"—
existing problem areas and predictable problems—before they surprise you at conversion.

While most hospitals understand the need for (and under-
estimate the time involved in) building order sets and cleaning up
their catalog, many have little appreciation for workflow. Often,
the hesitancy or aversion to workflow study reflects a distaste for
Visio diagrams and other arcane approaches to what is—in essence
at least—a simple issue. At its heart, the issue is not triangles,
squares, arrows, and diagrams, nor is it really arcane at all. The
issue is entirely concrete: It boils down to the perennial problem at
conversion, when the doctor or nurse, in a mix of frustration and

confusion, has no idea what to do. At its simplest, therefore, work-flow could merely consist of a series of questions and answers:

Q: Who puts in the "reason for visit"?
A: *The triage nurse.*
Q: Who is responsible for the transfer meds rec?
A: *The transferring physician.*
Q: Where does the paper EKG go when it's been done?
A: *In the boxes above the desk.*
Q: How long does a downtime have to be before we can just leave all the documentation on paper?
A: *Two hours.*

DEFINITION

Workflow is the daily, practical knowledge of how you perform patient care and how it will change with conversion. For example, workflow tells me how to admit patients; how to find an EKG; how to arrange a consult; how to get patients to radiology; and how to get patients out of their beds and home with all of their prescriptions, instructions, and follow-up arrangements. You may

---

A Poor Choice for Backups

One new hospital with an excellent EHR wasn't thoughtful enough about its workflow. Realizing that its EHR might occasionally fail, the hospital carefully developed an extensive and carefully planned "downtime policy," accompanied by all the backup forms needed for ordering and documenting if the computer were to fail.

It saved all of this material in its computer.

Which went down.

---

use a computer to perform these various functions, but workflow maps out the job and tells you **how** to use the computer when you perform them. If the computer is your clinical tool, then workflow is what you do with that tool in the day-to-day, nitty-gritty world of patient care.

If the EHR is a car, and training tells you how to start the car and use the pedals and gauges, then workflow tells you how to actually drive the car safely and efficiently. Clinical workflows are the shared assumptions about how we drive without hurting one another.

The best of cars can't make up for a bad driver. If we use the analogy of the EHR as a new car and the physician as the driver, then workflow is the collected rules of the road. It's as though we gave everyone in a town a new car, and the old rules—how we rode our horses around the town—might be adapted but are no longer sufficient. We need to decide hundreds of things that must become second nature. Which side of the road do we drive on? Do we stop at red lights? Can we turn right on red? Who has the right of way when I turn left across traffic? These questions are analogous to the workflow questions that arise when we "drive" an EHR: Which physician does the medication reconciliation? Can we override a drug allergy? Can we modify a drug order, or do we have to reorder it? Who writes the pain med orders in the PACU, and do these orders remain in effect once the patient has been transferred to an inpatient floor? These "rules of the road" are behavioral rather than electronic, processes rather than software, policies rather than computer limitations.

Many users think workflow is a waste of time. They feel that they already know what they do and that they will continue to do the same work after conversion. In reality, much of what they do will change, sometimes dramatically. Moreover, much of what they do now consists of informal policy exceptions, workarounds, and "understandings about how things are done here." In many cases, what policy explicitly spells out and what is actually done on the wards are different, sometimes shockingly so.

The essence of doing workflow is not so much defining what is "right" as discovering what is really being done and what works and then ensuring that it will still work when it is done on the computer.

The best software will fail if the workflow is wrong (and vice versa). Consider an example. In one hospital, the ICU policy clearly specified that vital signs must be taken every few minutes, but the nurses—finding it impossible to meet the policy and still care for patients—had a quiet understanding as to how often this task should actually be done. As we looked at the ICU workflow, even before adding in computers and bedside monitoring devices we found two disparate versions: the workflow specified in the written hospital policy and the real-life workflow of the ICU. As we designed the ICU order sets, we had to pick which of these two workflows—which frequency of vital signs—to use as an actual order. Until this point, the hospital had hummed along nicely despite the complete lack of connection between policy and reality. With the advent of the computer and the ability to measure actual compliance with hospital policy, the nurses would be forced to comply with whatever policy we chose. We could either change the policy to reflect a perhaps more realistic clinical practice (require vital signs to be taken less frequently) or force the nurses to comply with the more demanding clinical policy (require vital signs to be taken every few minutes). The underlying issue needed to be resolved: Was the policy unrealistic, or were the nurses not meeting a necessary standard? In short, policy and reality were about to become one, and we had to choose between them.

This sort of disparity—policy versus reality—is common in trivial matters and occasionally exists in more critical issues. Sometimes official policy is well intentioned but unrealistic, and reality is more appropriate. More commonly, policy is realistic and reality is inappropriate. In either case, the use of computer systems often requires us to discover what is actually occurring, compare it to what we want to achieve, and resolve the inconsistency to create a viable workflow. The advent of tasking, computerized monitoring, timed documentation, and clinical data mining make it impossible to sweep inconsistencies under the rug. We suddenly discover that our hospitals have been doing things that we didn't believe were happening and that we never would have sanctioned. In this sense, implementing a computer system allows us to reevaluate our clinical workflow and clean house.

Implementing a computer EHR is like turning over a rock.

TIMING

Workflows cannot be done at the last minute; they must be ready prior to training. Not only do we need the workflows to train clinical personnel; if we don't understand the workflows, we can't make the right decisions about how to build the system. We need to have a clear idea of what we are going to **do** with the system.

How patients will be admitted from the ED, for example, has practical consequences for the design of virtual beds, the initiation of orders, and registration's access privileges. To some extent, this situation becomes a catch-22: We can't define the future workflow without knowing how the system will be built, but we can't make the best decisions about how to build the system without understanding the workflow. Workflows and design decisions must go hand in hand. For most hospitals, the reality is that definition of workflow begins as early as possible, informs design decisions, and is complete prior to user training.

No matter how much care is put into mapping out workflows, however, they always will need to be fine-tuned after implementation. In fact, the best hospitals will continue to reevaluate and optimize both their order sets and their workflows on a regular basis, long after implementation. Both order sets and workflows are dynamic processes that must be adapted to changing technology, changing regulations, and changing medical care.

METHODS

Regardless of how we analyze workflows, the outcome is roughly equivalent as far as the clinical users are concerned: They learn what they should do (and not do) after conversion. The conversation often falls into a regular pattern: Here's what you should stop doing, here's what you should start doing, and here's what you should continue doing. Stop-start-continue training can be delivered through Visio diagrams or simply a long list of clinical behaviors in a Word document or on a spreadsheet.

The value of detailed studies—including Visio diagrams—lies in gaining a clear understanding of the totality of patient flow so

---

Examples of Workflow Questions

- When the ED physician documents that a patient will be admitted and signs the note, does that action automatically admit the patient, or does the physician need to place a separate order for the admission?
- During downtimes, where does the doctor find lab orders?
- After a medical code, do all the orders have to be entered into the computer?
- What ED documents (e.g., for child abuse, dog bites) will remain on paper?
- Can a physician log on to two computers at once?
- For documentation, can physicians share macros?
- Can we still register an unconscious trauma patient as "John Doe"?
- Where will I find radiology "wet reads"?
- If the nurse put doctor A's name on a triage protocol order but doctor B ended up seeing the patient, who actually signs the orders, and how?

---

that the answers to questions about workflow are accurate and complete. By themselves, the studies are of little value to the user, who merely wants to know what to do next—but they underlie and support the validity of the answers and guide training and policy.

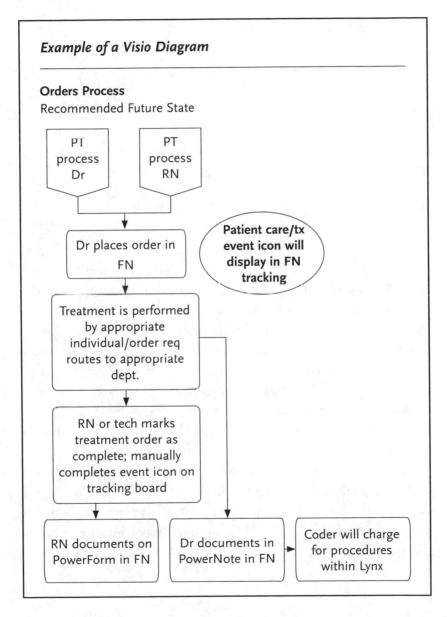

Example of a Visio Diagram

Orders Process
Recommended Future State

PT process Dr

PT process RN

Dr places order in FN

Patient care/tx event icon will display in FN tracking

Treatment is performed by appropriate individual/order req routes to appropriate dept.

RN or tech marks treatment order as complete; manually completes event icon on tracking board

RN documents on PowerForm in FN

Dr documents in PowerNote in FN

Coder will charge for procedures within Lynx

The key commonality is that at the time of conversion, no one should be wondering what to do. If the workflows are done well and user training is based on the workflows, clinical personnel never should have to ask:

- Where do I put the EKG?
- How do I admit the patient?
- Who initiates the orders?
- Do I print the discharge instructions?
- How do I arrange a consult?

Workflows feed into training, and training tells users not merely how to use a computer but also **what to do**.

WHERE ARE THE WORKFLOW ISSUES?

Workflow issues occur everywhere but are especially critical (and more numerous) wherever the patient changes venue. If we list several hundred workflow issues, almost all of them occur as the patient is admitted, moves from the ED to an inpatient floor, transfers into and out of the ICU, moves into and out of the operating room, moves through the PACU, or is discharged from the hospital. Given that physicians, locations, and orders can change rapidly, the PACU is usually a prime example of where to look carefully at workflow. Whenever the patient moves, things go wrong. Where these risks occur, it becomes imperative that we clarify what **should** happen if we are to deliver quality patient care.

The most common—and probably the best—way to organize workflow evaluations is to start from the beginning (the patient arrives at the hospital) and work through everything that happens to the patient until the end of the hospital stay (the patient leaves the hospital). There is no such thing as too much attention to workflow detail.

The biggest problems are always hidden in the questions you didn't ask. Inherent in every workflow session are issues of policy and protocol. If the nurse is to initiate orders, for example, does the nurse have the legal right (and the software privileges) to do so? The final workflow must reflect the hospital's policies and standard nursing and medical protocols, state licensing laws, Joint Commission policies, and currently accepted standards of medical care. Moreover, if we agree to change to a new workflow, and the clinical staff agree that the new workflow is medically appropriate but the current hospital policy differs from the new workflow, the current policy needs to be updated to reflect the new workflow. For example, if the policy states that the physician is to "sign the paper chart" but the workflow specifies electronic signature of the computer record, it is time to update the policy rather than construct an outdated workflow.

A Surprise to All

An ED with a volume of 100,000 patients per year had just converted to CPOE. The head physician saw his first patient, ordered a complete blood count (CBC) and an X-ray, and then walked over to the central work area to sit down and document the encounter. In his own words, here's what happened next: "Before I got my fanny on the chair, the radiology tech came in to take the patient for an X-ray. In 20 years, I'd never seen that happen before. The nurses always drew the blood, then it always took another 30 or 40 minutes before radiology showed up. Yet here he was, about to take her away, and we hadn't even drawn any blood. It sounds odd, but we had to figure out how to slow down radiology so that the nurses had time to get the blood draw."

Admissions—whether from the ED or directly to the inpatient floor—pose predictable workflow issues. The most common is: Who enters the list of the patient's home medications in the computer? This issue becomes particularly pressing not only because the admission medication reconciliation (meds rec) depends on having an accurate medications list but also because much of the patient's medical history is derived from knowledge of the patient's current medications. Knowing a patient is taking 120 mg of Lasix per day is much more useful and specific than knowing the patient has a history of hypertension. Having an "unclean" medications history creates extra work for physicians during meds rec and could mislead the treating physician when he is making important clinical decisions.

The process of entering medications into a computer can be time consuming, especially the first time it is done. This issue has prompted some hospitals to assign the task by venue (the data are entered by the ED nurse rather than by the triage nurse) or divide it between the two venues (the triage nurse enters the first half-dozen medications, and then the ED nurse finishes the rest of the list), but these approaches can produce errors and delays (to say nothing of finger-pointing). Another approach has been to assign the task to a pharmacist or a pharmacy technician, but this option can be too expensive or otherwise impractical, particularly in small community hospitals during night shifts and weekends, when pharmacy support is not cost-effective. In some hospitals, the job finally devolves to the physician, to the consternation of the medical staff.

The answer to the question of who should enter the patient's medication history (not the reconciliation) in the system should consider overall work efficiency; the job should not just be shifted to the physician (or the nurse). Regardless of the solution, a clearly mapped workflow will minimize any resultant problems.

General rule of workflow: Don't just shift work from physician to nurse or vice versa. Another common, almost universal workflow issue occurs in the ED when an admitted patient has to wait for a floor bed. Typically, the emergency physician has finished treating the patient, and the patient is relatively stable but is still occupying the gurney in the ED. A hospitalist comes down to the ED to write the inpatient orders. While the hospitalist wants a few stat orders done in the ED, he also places a number of orders meant to be done in the inpatient setting. If all the orders are acted on in the ED, not only will the ED nurses be tasked with jobs that aren't meant for them, but the pharmacy may well send the patient's drugs to the wrong unit (ED versus floor) and the orders may be billed for incorrectly (potentially putting the hospital at risk of being accused of billing fraud). The usual workflow solution (often involving "virtual" beds in the ED) is to carefully divide the two sorts of orders—stat ED orders versus floor orders—and ensure that the hospitalists, ED nurses, and pharmacy are entirely clear on which orders are for which venue. **When ED patients are waiting for a bed, always separate their stat orders from their floor orders.**

Transfers within a hospital create several predictable issues. The PACU is a common crossroads and—like any crossroads or roundabout—requires some attention to traffic flow. In general, the workflow of any PACU has evolved organically and has come to meet the needs of the clinical staff as they move patients from the operating room to the PACU and onto the floor. Nonetheless, these well-adapted workflows need to be explored for any changes inherent in the computer world. The two most common issues are: (1) Who writes the orders? and (2) Who does the meds rec? The answer to the first of these questions is established in every PACU, but with the advent of CPOE, there are new wrinkles, such as: Who cancels previous orders? For example, if a patient has a current order for a parenteral opiate drip, it may (in the paper world) be cancelled "automatically" when the patient leaves the PACU. In the computer world, however, the order must be actively cancelled. The answer might be that such orders are cancelled by protocol (the system), by a nurse, or by one of the physicians, but the answer must meet legal requirements, regulatory stipulations, and hospital policy. More important in purely **practical** terms, the clinical staff must clearly understand and accept the new workflow.

The issue of who does the meds rec is not limited to the PACU but is ubiquitous wherever transfers occur. Transferring patients into or out of the ICU, for example, always raises the same question. Ethically and medically, the responsibility is shared: Both the sending and the receiving physicians are equally responsible for providing good patient care and for ensuring that the medications—and indeed, all the orders—are appropriate and up to date. Practically, however, there is usually one of two normative answers to this question. The most common answer is that the receiving physician assumes the onus of care and takes responsibility for the meds rec. Whether the patient is transferring into or out of the ICU, the receiving physician—in this case the intensivist and the floor physician, respectively—completes this process. The second most common answer is that the onus is assumed by the physician at the higher level of care. In this case, whether the patient is transferring into or out of the ICU, the intensivist would complete the process.

Transfer meds rec raises another question: When do we need to do one at all? In the case of the ICU, the answer is considered obvious, but what about minor procedures? While a patient going from the floor to the operating room for an appendectomy is clearly being transferred, is a patient having an endoscopy considered a transfer? What about a patient who is having a pacemaker placed in the cardiology suite? What about a patient having a simple fluoroscopy-assisted lumbar puncture in radiology? What is needed is a simple, universal, unambiguous rule that the clinical staff can rely on, regardless of the time of day, the condition of the patient, or the physician involved. In many hospitals, the rule is that a transfer meds rec is required anytime a patient moves through the operating room but not for any other procedure location. Certainly, other rules can be (and have been) made, but this one provides a fairly clear definition: **Patients going through the operating room or the ICU require a transfer meds rec; other patients don't.**

Discharge also raises workflow problems. Most are minor and easily resolved, such as who prints the paperwork for the patient, who selects the patient instructions (doctor or nurse), or where to put paper prescriptions (if not using ePrescribe). More pressing problems involve the discharge meds rec and the problem of nursing home (or similar) transfers at discharge.

In the case of meds rec at discharge, the problem is not new but is newly highlighted. If an orthopedist is discharging a patient who has a new artificial hip, the orthopedist does not want to take responsibility for the several cardiac medications—medications that the orthopedist neither uses nor recognizes—at the time of discharge. Before hospitals had computers, the orthopedist would either call the cardiologist for advice or simply tell the patient to resume all prior medications but to check with his cardiologist. Both of these options are still available, but many specialists are leery of potential litigation when the electronic record seems to imply that they are prescribing medications they don't use or understand—even when the patient is simply resuming prior medications, as has always been done in the past. This concern has prompted many hospitals to add a disclaimer to the discharge instructions, warning patients to resume prior medications unless instructed otherwise but to follow up with their prescribing physicians.

There are two other common solutions, both involving the ability to do an electronic meds rec. The first solution is to have the admitting physician call various consultants and then do the discharge meds rec on the basis of their phone discussion (often called a "complete" meds rec). This solution implies that the admitting physician is "the captain of the ship," which is consistent with much of standard medical culture and policy. The second solution is to require each physician who is actively involved in the patient's care to participate in the discharge meds rec (often called a "partial" meds rec). The orthopedist reviews the orthopedic medications, the cardiologist reviews the cardiology medications, and so forth. In this solution, there is no single captain directing the meds rec, but medical care is considered a shared responsibility apportioned by specialty. The problem with the latter approach is tracking down the physicians who have completed the meds rec process and finding out when the patient is finally ready for discharge.

The physicians responsible for completing the discharge meds rec must be clearly spelled out.

During the discharge meds rec process, a common concern is defaulted orders and their implications for workflow versus risk. In the case of discharge medications, most patients will resume most of their prior home medications and will stop taking their inpatient hospital medications. Because this order is most commonly selected, many EHRs offer the option of setting it as a default: The home medications order defaults to "cancel hospital medications and resume prior home medications." The discharging physician then reviews and corrects the default list to accord with the actual medical intent.

While some hospitals decry the risk of inadvertently prescribing an unnecessary medication (or inadvertently not prescribing a necessary one), the benefits to physician workflow (e.g., time savings) gained by defaulting this choice are enormous. Likewise, not using the default option carries the risk of prescription errors. As always, there is a delicate balance between the interests of workflow—how to get things done efficiently—and risk—how to get things done safely.

The final common discharge problem is that of transfer to another facility, such as a skilled nursing facility, nursing home, rehabilitation facility, or tertiary care hospital. In this case, the patient isn't staying in the hospital, nor is he going home. The discharging physician does not want responsibility for writing the prescriptions—because he will not be treating the patient—but he does want to indicate his recommended treatment. Many current EHR vendors—and many workflows—fail to take this common practice into account. The patient should leave not only with clear suggestions (not prescriptions) for recommended therapy but also with a medical summary. This summary must often be tailored to the needs of the receiving facility and is by no means the same as the standard patient instructions or the standard medical discharge summary.

All of the discussion thus far has concerned inpatient workflow. The ambulatory setting also has its own native problems. One common thread is that hospital workflows are not readily translated into ambulatory workflows. Many hospitals assume RNs perform certain tasks (e.g., obtaining the medication list) when in ambulatory clinics these tasks are often done by medical assistants. Speed is an issue: The physician barks out orders in rapid succession as he exits the exam room, and procedure and billing codes must be entered immediately (rather than days or weeks later, as is typical of inpatient care). Furthermore, a bill must be produced at checkout so that copayments and charges are dealt with before the patient leaves the office. All of these items may be difficult to capture/produce efficiently when CPOE and computer scheduling are required. These tasks are especially difficult when a system does not support future orders (e.g., a repeat CBC in four weeks and another chest X-ray in six months) or required information is not readily available (e.g., a future encounter number). Phoned-in refill requests add to the potential confusion. All of these processes must be carefully planned out and adapted to changing workflows as the clinic transitions to a fully computerized practice.

In all cases, the rule of thumb remains constant: **The starting point for implementing any workflow is its current state.** Begin with the usual workflow, and adapt it as needed.

Any workflow session begins with the same question: What do you currently do? Other things being equal, the workflow should remain unchanged; the easiest workflow to manage is the one that is the same as it used to be. There are only two reasons to change an old workflow. The first reason is that the computer supports a different workflow. If it's easier, faster, and legally appropriate to sign charts electronically, why should we keep signing them with a pen? The second reason is that we discover (sometimes to our surprise and horror) that the old workflow was inappropriate or even dangerous. Implementation then becomes a chance to clean house. In the ideal world, workflows change because the new workflow is either easier or safer.

WHO DOES WORKFLOW?

Putting it practically, workflows are generally defined by a location (e.g., PACU, ED, operating room, labor and delivery), not by a position (e.g., physician, nurse, pharmacist). The people involved in a particular workflow are those who work together in a common venue. For example, the standard workflow of a physician in the PACU involves not only surgeons and anesthesiologists but also the PACU nurses, the PACU secretary, respiratory technicians, radiologists, the pharmacy, the lab, and others. This same rule pertains to any location: Workflows describe the activity of people who work together in a common area.

Never Cut a Single Workflow into Two Separate Workflows

The PACU staff of a busy urban hospital used a two-sided "pink form," with one side for doctors' information and the other side for nurses' information. The physicians didn't talk to the nurses who, prior to conversion, had translated their side of the form into the computer and then removed the paper form from the PACU, assuming they would no longer need it. Likewise, the nurses didn't talk to the physicians, who had simply assumed that they would keep using the paper form because no one had said otherwise. On the morning of the conversion, surgery ground to a halt when the physicians discovered that the paper form was gone and there was no corresponding physician form available in the computer.

Workflow sessions are a team sport; they involve everyone who plays a role in treating patients in the location of the workflow and anyone who interfaces with those treating the patient. In a usual workflow session, input is required not only from the physicians and nurses involved but also often from the pharmacists and, depending on what questions come up, from other personnel, including dietitians, registration staff, respiratory and physical therapists, and whoever else has an impact on patient care in that location. In addition, workflows are usually—and appropriately—reviewed by those addressing quality assurance or regulatory concerns for the hospital.

WORKFLOW DISRUPTION

Not all changes are equal. Depending on what is being implemented, the degree to which workflow will be disrupted by conversion differs markedly, as does the amount of effort that should be spent on defining and plotting out the workflows in a hospital. If we divide the implementation of medical systems into (1) viewing results, (2) placing orders, and (3) documenting, disruption of physician workflow increases as we progress through these stages.

In general, viewing medical data—labs, documents, and so on—in the computer is relatively easy to learn and occasions little change in the workflow of most physicians. They find that viewing data in a computer is simple and intuitive, even if they have not grown up using computers. Equally, even the most curmudgeonly of older physicians is happy to be able to sign charts and orders by accessing the medical records at his desk rather than by walking down to the medical records department to find and physically thumb through charts. Viewing (and electronic signing) is not markedly disruptive to physician workflow.

Placing orders is another matter. Many current CPOE interfaces are awkward and involve unnecessary clicking and scrolling, and physicians must be trained to use them. And these technicalities are not the only stress-inducing factors during a CPOE conversion. The workflow itself is necessarily changed, partly as a result of the need to log on, and the brunt of the stress falls on physicians who place "serial" rather than "parallel" orders. In the paper world, there is little difference between serial and parallel orders from the physician's perspective, but to place serial orders in the computer world—that is, order a first test, then later a second test, and finally a third test—the physician has to log on and access the ordering interface three separate times. To place parallel orders—that is, order all three tests at once—the physician has to log on only once. The upshot is that physicians who habitually place their orders serially find their workflow is disrupted significantly, more so than the workflow of physicians who naturally place their orders in parallel. For almost all physicians, the result is a moderate change in how they see their patients: CPOE is somewhat disruptive to physician workflow.

Documenting is, oddly enough, the most likely task to cause stress and disrupt physician workflow, partly because of the interface used to document on a computer, but not entirely so. Even the advantages of computer documentation—such as the ability to document piecemeal rather than needing to dictate the entire patient note at one time—change the way the physician sees patients and are inherently disruptive of the pre-conversion workflow. Moreover, documentation now may be completed earlier in patient encounters, and emphasis may be placed on different goals (e.g., the increased emphasis on regulatory compliance, structured history, coding of diagnoses).

In any project in which workflow is being evaluated, the amount of effort and time required to get the workflow right will, roughly speaking, reflect all the considerations we have just discussed. The viewing of medical data in a computer requires little consideration of workflow changes, CPOE requires that a great deal of thought be given to workflow changes, and computer documentation—whether using electronic templates, word recognition software, or both—requires at least as much attention to workflow changes as does CPOE.

KEY POINTS

- Workflows tell users exactly what to do at conversion.
  - —Completed workflows are required for both training and conversion.
  - —Visio diagrams, Excel spreadsheets, or Word documents can be used to map out workflows.
  - —The outcome is a clear set of guidelines on how to proceed.
- Workflows are defined by places and patients, not by position.
  - —Watch for issues when a patient changes status or changes venue.
  - —Common locations include such venues as the ED, operating room, PACU, and labor and delivery.
  - —Most workflows include physicians, nurses, and pharmacists, as well as other personnel.
- Caveats and predictable issues include the following:
  - —Admission, transfers, and discharges pose predictable workflow issues.
  - —Which physicians are responsible for meds rec?
  - —Ambulatory workflow has its own separate issues.
  - —CPOE and computer documentation are more disruptive to physician workflow than is viewing data.

CHAPTER 7

Communication and Training

*I never teach my pupils; I only attempt to provide
the conditions in which they can learn.*

—*Albert Einstein*

IN THE RUN-UP to conversion, communication and training often receive short shrift. They tend to be the "neglected stepchildren" of the project. They aren't more important than any of the previously discussed material, but they are equal partners in the success of any implementation. Just as projects fail as a result of poor governance, a faulty catalog, or neglected workflows, they fail if communication and training are ignored, delayed, or mismanaged.

In a hospital implementation, success depends on parts of the project working together—not only the "brain" of good governance but all of the "organs" of the project, including training and communication.

TIMING

Most project decisions affect training, and training has implications for the rest of the project. Too often, trainers are brought in four weeks prior to conversion and asked to simply "teach the system." While the training itself should be scheduled as close as possible to the conversion, **preparations** for that training need to be made as early as possible in the project calendar. The major considerations are

1. adapting the training to the hospital's culture, policies, and computer domains;
2. coordinating the trainers, the users, and their positions; and
3. having a realistic understanding of training costs and infrastructure.

Consider the analogy of driving a car: Training people to drive is not simply a matter of teaching them how to start the car and use the controls; they also must learn the rules of the road and safe-driving techniques and become familiar with some of the local terrain. Training physicians and nurses to use an EHR is much the same: They need to understand their hospital's policies, their workflows, and how their specific build and domain will work as they deliver medical care. Not only will trainers need to have access to (and an understanding of) the final decisions regarding policies, workflow, and build; they also will need to provide feedback on what can be most easily taught and remembered so that reasonable modifications to the policies, workflow, and build can be made if necessary. Complex policies are difficult to teach and almost impossible to remember. Project decisions need to reflect the limitations and norms of human behavior. We should not teach policies that staff will never follow. The upshot is simple: Involve trainers early and completely. When you plan the project, plan the training.

COMMUNICATION

Communication deserves the same care as training. Communication begins with the initiation of the project. From the moment you know the answer to the question "Why are we doing this?" you should communicate it to everyone, involved or not, and without delay. If you are implementing an EHR to improve patient care, tell your employees and make sure they understand this rationale before you begin. In an EHR implementation, there is no such thing as communicating too early or offering people too much information when they want it.

In communications, the value of honesty cannot be overstated. When you hide facts, people assume the worst. When you gloss over the bad aspects, people stop believing the good aspects. Communicate your problems, your concerns, and even your failures. The best way to build credibility is to admit error, without exaggeration and without attempting to evade responsibility.

Self-deprecation is endearing; credibility is earned by being open and honest.

Tell the Truth, or Gossip Wins

In one large chain of hospitals, administrators gave staff no information whatsoever regarding the rationale for the upcoming implementation, nor did they provide their criteria for choosing a vendor. If clinical personnel had been consulted, none of the staff knew who might have been involved in the decision.

The total communication vacuum was immediately filled by gossip.

An early rumor circulated, and it became "common knowledge" that the vendor was chosen solely because the CIO's brother-in-law (who worked for the vendor) had talked him into buying an unnecessary, second-rate system. Clearly, patient care, ease of use, and other considerations had been sacrificed to nepotism, and the staff became furious.

Once the rumor began, no amount of belated communication or goodwill was able to overcome the staff's belief that they had been "sold out." A decade later, many of the staff still believe the rumor.

How to Communicate

Communication is not only what you say but also what others hear.

More accurately, the critical feature is what the other party understands. This concept applies equally when the communication is written and read. The ultimate question is not the intent but the outcome.

In discussions about communication, an understandable emphasis is placed on learning to express oneself clearly. Certainly the first two steps involved in successful communication are to (1) have a clear understanding of what you are trying to say—that is, thinking clearly and organizing your thoughts, and (2) express those thoughts clearly and unambiguously. Both of these skills—thinking well and speaking well—are required foundations for communication. However, communication is not one-way; it involves two parties and should be reciprocal. The reciprocal steps are the second two requirements for any successful communication: (1) The listener must accurately understand what you meant (not what you said), and (2) the speaker should confirm that understanding. Anything short of this dialogue may result in good communication, but only as a matter of luck and guesswork.

How Not to Communicate

Often, failure results solely because the speaker hasn't considered the context of the listener. The most common example is the use

---

Four Requirements of Successful Communication

1. Clear **thinking** by the speaker.
2. Clear **expression** by the speaker.
3. Accurate **understanding** by the listener.
4. **Confirmation** of the listener's understanding.

---

of jargon and abbreviations. The speaker assumes that his jargon is understood; the listener is lost and often unwilling to admit her ignorance.

If you are addressing people in another time zone, don't assume they know which one you are in. When you ask, "Can you be on a call at 4 p.m.?" do you mean Alaska time, Atlantic time, or one of the time zones between those two?

Communicating Nonsense

In this actual e-mail, notice that the sender assumed— incorrectly, as it turned out—that the recipient would know which notifications, which documents, which choices, and which groups she was referring to:

> Subject: Please Turn Off E-mail Notifications for the Morning of 4/25/12
>
> Hello,
>
> I will be creating several new documents in this group, and when you create a new document, you are not given the choice of minor edit, do not publish, so I would recommend turning off all e-mail notifications from this group for the remainder of the morning.
>
> Thanks

The recipient had never heard of the sender and had not the slightest idea of what she was referring to, and—as a direct result—the e-mail was incomprehensible. Moreover, the recipient wasted half an hour checking whether the e-mail referred to items that required action on his part. It did not.

This communication not only failed but also wasted time and resources.

If you work in more than one hospital, don't assume that the listener knows which hospital you are talking about. The question "Can you work a shift on Saturday?" does not provide enough detail. At which hospital? On which unit in that hospital?

If you use an abbreviation, make sure the listener uses the same abbreviation. You may think the question "What do you think about the MS?" is clear enough—but are you talking about multiple sclerosis, mental status, morphine sulfate, mitral stenosis, or something else?

Communications Team

A communications team or an individual who "drives" communications is assigned to most projects to ensure fluid exchange both from the project team to the entire hospital staff and—less often, but important—from the hospital staff back to the project team. Communication venues vary widely as our culture transitions from the world of letters, faxes, and telephones to the world of e-mail, texting, and social networks. The use of cell phones and hospital websites are as important as posters and notices placed in wards or in the physicians' lounge.

The wide variety of communication methods—and the fact that some physicians refuse to use certain methods—makes communication difficult, but the very breadth of options may help ensure that the messages get through to their targets. If you don't use e-mail, I can call your office; if you don't like faxes, I can text you; if you never come to our staff meetings, I can use LinkedIn; if you don't see the poster in the physicians' lounge, I can buttonhole you in the hall. Most venues for communication not only are in flux but also have wildly different patterns of usage, loosely correlating with the age of the user. **Communicate not by a single method but by all available methods.**

Communication is not limited to the hospital staff; it must include patients, their families, all other visitors, and the broader community and catchment area of the hospital. These people are the hospital's "customers," and while they may not be using the EHR, they need to understand the implications of EHR use for their hospital experience and for any patient visit. Those visiting the hospital should receive a message that stresses the hospital's desire to deliver improved patient care focused on quality, compassion, speed, and safety issues. The key message is often modified to accord with recent Press Ganey scores or other information regarding what the community or the patient base perceives as either weak points or important features that distinguish local hospitals. With these points in mind, the hospital needs to create both an internal and an external plan for communications at the onset of the project. The plan should represent input from clinical staff and the clinical education and hospital public relations (or marketing) departments.

OVERVIEW OF TRAINING

Training poses three recurrent, predictable, and preventable problems:

1. It isn't clinical.
2. It isn't sufficient.
3. It isn't provided in time.

The results are failed workflow, markedly unhappy clinical personnel, and increased patient risks.

Training Must Be Clinical

The single most common failure of training is an emphasis on "button pressing" rather than on treating patients. As an example, consider teaching surgeons to order blood products:

- Poor training consists of showing the surgeons how to find the order set for blood products (how to search the name of the order set, how to choose the orderables needed, and so on) and then place the orders.

- Optimal training places the order for blood products in a realistic clinical context: The surgeon is given an example of a patient who is exsanguinating (e.g., a trauma patient or a patient with gastrointestinal bleeding), and—as part of the appropriate sequence of clinical actions—the surgeon is encouraged to give packed red blood cells.

A similar failure occurs when physicians are trained to use macros in documentation. The actual skill of constructing and saving macros is mindlessly simple, but the essential clinical perspective consists of knowing which macros to construct and how those macros increase the efficiency and safety of caring for patients in a real clinical situation. Any trainer can explain the use of macros, but a clinical perspective is required to understand the need for layered macros (which progressively hone in on findings) and procedure macros (which are tailored to the individual physician's practice preferences). **Training physicians to press buttons is training for project failure. Train clinically.**

Not only is clinically based training easier to get across to users; their retention is longer lasting, and the day of conversion is far less stressful. The implication is that optimal training requires that trainers have a clinical background. The best trainers are those who have experience in the same settings where staff work. In general, the most useful and most successful trainers are physicians and nurses, who not only appreciate workflow issues but also can train in a clinical context. Physicians make especially good trainers because their workflow is inherently focused not on specific actions but on decision making that prompts clinical actions. The essence of a physician's job is not ordering blood but rather deciding whether to order blood and only then taking action (or not). Training that emphasizes action without reference to the decision-making process is unnatural and counterproductive. **Effective trainers must have clinical experience.**

Training Must Be Sufficient

The second most common error is insufficient training. The error here is not simply the amount of training but also the quality and sequence of training. Optimal training requires that the user understand not only the interface—in a clinical context—but also the changes in policies, processes, and workflow that are inherent in converting to an EHR. Moreover, there is a natural sequence to such training: It starts with fundamental issues (e.g., access to the computer, navigation of the screens), progresses to the daily "gist"

If You Require It, Say So

A small hospital on the East Coast was diligent about tracking those who had not been trained but did nothing to follow up and prod those individuals to get trained. Nor did it provide any impetus or explain the consequences of not being trained. The medical executive committee and the hospital board had unanimously agreed that physicians would be required to complete training to have clinical privileges, but this decision was not communicated to the training staff or the attending physicians.

At go-live, the hospital had trained less than 30 percent of its attending staff, predominantly the hospitalists, and was faced with a hospital policy that forbade untrained physicians to see patients. That morning, large numbers of nurses and physicians were told that they could not see patients, and almost all clinical care ground to a halt. An emergency meeting (of both the board and the medical executive committee) was called, the policy was postponed, training was enforced, and the situation slowly improved.

The hospital lost income for a few weeks and goodwill from both patients and clinical staff for a good several months.

---

of computer use (finding results, placing orders, and documenting), and—only after these initial skills are mastered—concludes with fine points and high-level skills. A common example is learning macros for clinical documentation; the physician first learns how to create macros and then later learns which macros are actually useful for documenting clinical care.

Learning advanced skills is difficult if you haven't actually used basic skills. While some training regimens attempt to pack both types of skills into a single sequence of classes, many successful projects use the "circle back" method: They train clinical personnel on all of the necessary skills for a successful implementation and then circle back a week (or six weeks) later to correct errors, fine-tune skills, and add the advanced skills that make the difference between grudging use of the computer and elegant, efficient use of the computer as a clinical tool.

The latter approach—circling back to complete training after initial conversion—has become more common and even recommended in recent years, although there is no consensus on how to handle the mechanics and scheduling of this process or on exactly which skills to include. Post-conversion training is also an appropriate time to assess and improve usage habits (e.g., building favorites and macros, sequential versus parallel ordering, coordinating results viewing with documentation) and to adjust filters, fonts, defaults, and all other user-based preferences. Even physicians who have used EHRs for years are often unaware of small tweaks that can be made to user preferences to enable more efficient, or simply more pleasant, use of the system.

Training Must Be Timed Appropriately

The third most common error is the timing (and organization) of the training. In the ideal world, training would occur immediately prior to the go-live date. However, any practical attempt to follow this ideal precept would result in disaster due to trying to schedule training for large numbers of hospital personnel. If a hospital has a medical staff of a thousand who are all going live Monday at 8 a.m., there is no possible way to train them all simultaneously Sunday evening. The practical precept is therefore more accommodating: **Training should occur as late as possible but early enough to get everyone trained.**

Saved at the Last Moment

A large, urban medical center was less than two months from conversion, and no one knew who had been trained, if anyone. The lead trainer had no plan, no syllabus, no list of physicians or nursing personnel at any of the center's eight hospital facilities, no defined deadlines, and no clear reporting line below him.

The CEO fired the lead trainer.

A vice president was placed in charge, along with a new director of medical informatics. Within days, they had an accurate database containing the names of all physician staff and their specialties, department chairs, office phones, cell phones, home phones, e-mail addresses, and training status. They had parallel information on the nursing staff, ward secretaries, and ancillary clinical staff, all of which was kept up to date. They created a firm training schedule, assigned deadlines and responsible parties, estimated costs, and identified backfill staffing needs. Training proceeded rapidly and effectively, and progress was tracked by logging which medical staff had (and hadn't) been trained, date of training (scheduled or completed), competency score, and whether remedial action was taken. Conversion went ahead on schedule with unequaled physician adoption relative to that at other hospitals. All eight hospitals became a model for other implementation projects.

But it is not that simple: The precept assumes that trainers, rooms, and computers are available and that we have some flawless way of making appointments, following up on those who missed training, and keeping a precise and accurate record of who was (and wasn't) trained, plus a plan for mitigating the number of "escapees" from training.

Sufficient training has three components: (1) a tight, clinically based syllabus, (2) a clinically based test of competency, and (3) an accurate method of tracking students and trainers.

PLANNING DETAILS FOR SUCCESSFUL TRAINING

For a training plan to be successful, three components must be precisely defined at the onset:

1. The syllabus for each training session
2. The hours needed per training session
3. The resources necessary for training

The material that staff are required to learn is delineated in the syllabus and varies by position. The number of hours required to learn the material also vary by position and—to some extent—by the previous experience of the staff member. Required resources include classrooms, computers, super-users, trainers, backfill staff (for those being trained), money, and basic infrastructure.

Syllabus

The training syllabus is defined by position. The most common distinction is that between the physician syllabus and the nursing syllabus, but similar distinctions must be made for the ward secretary, the pharmacist, the respiratory technician, the radiology technician, and other clinical positions. A few positions always are neglected—or totally forgotten—to the detriment of workflow at conversion. These positions are nonetheless important and include social workers, ministers, dietary workers, and so on. Each position has its own needs, workflows, and distinct syllabus.

The position defines the workflow; the workflow defines the syllabus. As pointed out in previous chapters, it is crucial that the workflows have been completely defined prior to training, including all policies and procedures, which often underlie and define the boundaries of a workflow. If a hospital hasn't decided how to handle standing orders, for example, there is no policy for nurses to learn. Even if we allow for the requirement that workflows be defined prior to training, the majority of workflows are not defined by policy decisions but by the nature of the position. Nursing workflows are, in general, well defined and largely invariant between hospitals, but they do vary between wards. While the typical nurse can move from one hospital's med-surg ward to another with a modicum of orientation, major differences are involved when a nurse changes positions, such as from a med-surg nurse to an operating room nurse. Workflows differ markedly by location in the hospital, and the syllabi need to reflect these differences as well as the clinical questions that those in each position typically have during training.

A typical syllabus begins with a simple vision statement explaining the rationale behind the conversion, gives a brief overview of the interface, and then delves into workflow specifics. In general, a good syllabus has two phases: The first shows how to do specific actions (e.g., how to order a gram of cefazolin), and the second places these actions in a clinical context (e.g., you have a sepsis patient who needs treatment, including an antibiotic such as cefazolin). The first phase is didactic and well defined, while the second phase is often more self-directed, giving the user a chance to explore the system, albeit with some help. A single trainer can deliver the first phase to numerous students, but the second phase requires a higher ratio of trainers to students, raising the obvious question of what that ratio should be. Not surprisingly, the answer varies for several reasons. The most common recommendation (more honored in the breach than the observance) is that all physician training be one on one, pairing a single trainer with each physician. This suggestion is becoming passé and probably resulted from various factors: Compared to typical trainees, physicians tend to be older (and often less computer savvy), have little patience for wasting time in classrooms, have a high cost per hour, and have limited available time (and even less scheduling flexibility). In reality, the ratio

---

Typical Questions That Underlie and Define a Physician Syllabus

- How do I find:
  - —The patient's laboratory data?
  - —The patient's X-ray, ultrasound, CT, and MRI views?
  - —The radiologist's reports?
  - —The patient's previous records?
- How do I sign or co-sign:
  - —My charts or dictations?
  - —The resident's charts or his/her orders?
- Where is my:
  - —Daily clinic schedule?
  - —Surgery schedule?
  - —On-call schedule?
- How do I document:
  - —Histories and physicals?
  - —Surgical notes?
  - —Progress notes?
- How do I obtain a consult?
- How do I place an order?
- How do order sets work?

---

of physicians to trainers can be higher in certain circumstances, such as for the training of residents (or medical students) who—compared to attending physicians—are more technologically savvy (i.e., younger), have a lower cost per hour, and have more flexible schedules. In many cases, the physician-to-trainer ratio also can be higher if the physicians share a single specialty (e.g., training five orthopedic surgeons simultaneously) or for the initial phase of training (as described earlier). From a purely practical perspective, ratios of up to a dozen attending physicians to one trainer are occasionally feasible and can achieve good outcomes if the training is done carefully and with strenuous attention to the different needs (and technological knowledge) of the individual physicians.

As a general rule, classroom ratios can be equally high (i.e., 12:1) or even higher for nurses and other personnel, again with due care that the individuals are actually learning the workflows and will be able to provide safe and efficient patient care. One problem in scheduling training for nursing staff is the requirement for (and cost of) backfilling their positions on the ward. Not only must the hospital pay to have the nurse sit in a classroom for training; an equivalent cost accrues when another nurse is paid to cover the clinical responsibilities of the first nurse. Not surprisingly, conflicts arise when a hospital tries to schedule 30 nurses for training while simultaneously trying to find another 30 nurses to take over their shifts. Once again, careful organization is required not only to schedule training but also to find and schedule additional nursing FTEs to fill the empty nursing slots created when nurses are in the classroom.

Whether for nurses or physicians, ratios of 30:1 are almost never recommended, except for orientation purposes (e.g., an introductory talk about the nature of training by the chief nursing officer or chief medical officer). In actual training, however, a typical set of normative values (averaging all cases) might suggest that in optimal circumstances, the physician-to-trainer ratio could be as high as 6:1, and for other clinical personnel, at least twice that (12:1).

Hours

The hours required for training vary enormously both within and between hospitals and are dictated by three factors:

1. The skills being taught (e.g., viewing data, CPOE, documentation)
2. The position or workflow (e.g., PACU nurse versus neurosurgeon)
3. The prior skills of the group or individual

In general, viewing data (e.g., finding a patient's laboratory results) requires the least training time (a few hours), while CPOE and documentation require substantially more training time (twice that needed for viewing data). With regard to position, nurses and physicians require approximately the same number of training hours, with exceptions imposed by their differing workflows. Certain nurses (e.g., in the ICU) may need to be trained to handle a bedside medical device interface, document a multiplicity of patient data, and do CPOE, while other nurses (e.g., in a med-surg ward) may not need the same complexity of training. Likewise, physicians differ in how (and the degree to which) they document on a day-to-day basis; some use an electronic template, some use word recognition software, and some use both. Whether physicians have these different skills varies depending on specialty, location, and type of workflow. Some physicians start with a broad base of technological skills from their daily life (e.g., texting, using smartphones, reading e-books, gaming, surfing the Internet), while others cling to paper, landlines, and libraries, disdaining (or fearing) computer access and the use of electronic media.

Given these caveats and concerns, there are guidelines for the number of hours required to provide basic training to most clinical staff:

- Data viewing: Two to four hours
- CPOE: Four to six hours

- Documentation: Four to six hours
- Word recognition: Two to four hours

These guidelines do not address, however, the use of "playtime," practice, or circling back to optimize use of the system. Learning how to create a macro, for example, requires only a few minutes; becoming adept at using macros may require days or weeks. The same is true of all of the training topics: Basic training is short; becoming adept is time consuming. In many cases, this additional time is incorporated into formal training, increasing the classroom time requirement. In other cases, this additional time is left informal and, while recommended, is not required.

Regardless of how formal or informal the training sessions may be, most hospitals require a competency assessment. It may be done informally (e.g., the trainer confirms that staff have successfully completed the sessions) or formally (e.g., staff take a computer-based exam). The informal option is more common, but there is a growing tendency toward requiring staff to pass a formal competency exam. A growing number of physicians and nurses have already been trained either at previous hospitals or during medical school, so some clinical personnel may not need formal training

---

Example of the Amount of Training per Physician at a Large Southern Academic Hospital

- Six hours total, split into two sessions:
    — Session 1 (three hours): CPOE, chart navigation, and workflow
    — Session 2 (three hours): documentation (by template), favorites, macros, autotext, pre-completed notes, meds reconciliation, and electronic prescribing
- Optional (two hours): Dragon training (see Chapter 3)

to pass the exam, except for sessions on hospital policies and local workflows. **Successful completion of competency exams may supersede the need for training, but policies and workflows must be taught.**

Resources

The syllabi and hours are the primary determinants of the resources required for an implementation, but the process is still complex and a surprise to many project planners. Training almost always takes more resources than are estimated, so careful budgeting and fore-thought are required.

As a rule, resources are estimated initially and then honed on the basis of actual numbers (e.g., trainers, trainees, domains, classrooms, computers, hours per trainee). Trainers are trained first, followed by super-users and then finally the remainder of the staff. Super-users serve two purposes. The primary intent is to provide support at the time of conversion because (1) they have extra training and (2) they are clinicians and thus best able to appreciate and support clinical users. The secondary intent is to provide public relations support to the clinical staff by "spreading the word" and allaying fears. In some systems, super-users also assist during staff training.

Who Provides the Training?

To define resource needs, the hospital has to decide who will provide the training. The vendor, a third-party company, or the hospital itself can fulfill this role. On the one hand, training uses an inordinate and often unprecedented number of resources, which argues in favor of bringing in outside training resources. On the other hand, an internal coterie of trainers can continue to provide expertise in the future, enabling rapid training of new personnel and flexible support for continuing staff needs.

Even if a hospital chooses to bring in an outside training group, it should ensure that the outside group provides special training to its own internal educators so that once the contract finishes, the hospital has a permanent set of internal training resources. These individuals do not have to be restricted to a training role alone; the best trainer resources are individuals who continue to provide clinical care and understand clinical workflow. Optimally, any hospital—after conversion—maintains a list of physicians, nurses, and pharmacists who have the additional qualification of being able to train future physicians, nurses, and pharmacists. This same group can function as a key set of personnel for later projects as well, such as when the hospital undertakes future advances in computer systems, and can serve on or provide input for standing committees that maintain and oversee order sets, hospital policies, and clinical decision-making tools.

Type of Training

Training can be done in any number of ways, but the most common pitfall is to try to deliver low-cost training by relying solely (or predominantly) on web-based or computer-assisted learning modules. While they can be effective (e.g., for introducing staff to the interface or teaching basic computer literacy), they are generally disappointing (or total failures) when used in a clinical context. Many hospitals successfully use web-based training as a do-it-yourself introduction and then follow up with classroom instruction in which a trainer is present to guide and assist those being trained. Successful training always has a strong element of personal contact in a classroom setting, with or without supplemental web-based training.

Informal training should occur concomitantly in staff meetings, sponsored events, and other contexts. While these venues generally are reserved for hospital and job-related communications, they equally are opportunities to teach. One of the most successful ways of ensuring adoption is to have trainers (or super-users) present tailored material at departmental or section meetings of the medical staff. Similar meetings work for nursing and other staff members and should be encouraged, if not made a formal part of the training plan.

If an outside group is used for training, be sure it uses web-based approaches appropriately (not solely) and takes advantage of informal opportunities to train your users.

Don't Ask; Do Tell

A Midwestern community hospital was afraid to make training mandatory for fear of alienating its staff. Moreover, given its lack of financial resources, the hospital opted to do without classroom training time and use web-based training exclusively. It was equally unwilling to pay the nursing (or physician) staff to complete the training, so clinical staff were told to do web-based training "whenever they have a bit of extra time."

Rarely do nurses or physicians have extra time. Even when not engaged in patient contact, they are absorbed by documentation and other demands. Informal staff surveys showed that staff universally felt the underlying message was that training was not important or even necessary.

At the time of conversion, less than 10 percent of the staff had spent time using the web-based training and not a single staff member had completed it.

Conversion was halted less than an hour after the system was turned on, and it was postponed for almost another year, resulting in significant financial loss.

Analysis of Training Needs

Needs analysis can be frightening, but it is necessary. Consider the needs of a moderate-sized community hospital that will implement CPOE and computer documentation for the nursing and physician staff. The following figures are drawn from an actual hospital but are given here for demonstration purposes only:

- Training software for CPOE and electronic documentation
- Training time per physician: 6 hours (approximate; ranges from 4 to 12 hours)
- Training time per nurse: 6 hours (approximate; ranges from 2 to 16 hours)
- Number of physician staff: 412
- Number of nurses and other clinical staff: 1,491
- Actual total hours: 12,352
- Training window: 7 weeks
- Seats per classroom: 8 to 12
- Class hours per day: 12 (3 hours per class)
- Classrooms available: 5
- Classes per week: 130 (some classes meet on weekends)
- Training domains: 1 (refreshed nightly)
- Super-users: 114
- Full-time trainers: 8

The implications are surprising to those not familiar with the training needs of hospitals. Not only does the hospital require eight FTE instructors (including salary and benefits); the total number of training hours (12,352) also has two financial implications: (1) The actual training time for clinical staff is the equivalent of more than six FTE nurses (and physicians), and (2) the equivalent of another six FTE nurses (and physicians) is needed to backfill the clinical time for those engaged in training. **Training is costly; it must be budgeted early and accurately.**

The costs involved in training do not end there. A training domain—essentially an accurate and functional copy of the final "prod" domain that will be used in clinical practice—must be available for use before the final domain goes live (with implications for deadlines and IT staffing) and be maintained and "kept clean" over the course of training. Moreover, any errors found in this domain must be corrected in real time or the training schedule will derail. A hospital cannot afford to have its training domain go down for a day. Not only will several classes have to be canceled as a result; some individuals may not be able to reschedule training before the go-live date, and potentially irreparable damage may be done to the credibility of the IT department when the clinical

---

Needs Versus Availability

The following tables compare the actual needs of a typical hospital (the number of hours it needed to train its nurses) and available resources (rooms, seats, and hours when nurses were available to be trained and could be back-staffed):

Required time resources:

Solution	Training Hours	Seats	Total Hours
System	2	984	1,968
Order set use	2	564	1,128
Nursing CPOE	1	524	524
Documentation	2	376	752

Available room resources:

Training Room	Number of Seats	Percentage Available	Hours/Day
Room A	13	80	12
Room B	8	100	12
Room C	8	100	12
Room TBD	8	100	12
Practice room	6	100	24

staff, not understanding the difference between the training and prod domains, come to believe that the domain doesn't work and is unsafe for patient care. A stable, reliable, accurate reflection of the final prod domain is necessary to provide accurate training and instill confidence in clinical users.

Offering Inducements and Motivating Users

In most hospitals, nursing staff are under contract and can be required to undergo training. While this requirement obligates the hospital to pay training costs, the issue of motivating nurses to complete training does not arise, or if it does arise, it is minor in comparison to the issue of motivating physicians. As a general rule—although it has been changing rapidly—hospitals do not reimburse physicians for their time in training. Contract physicians—typically hospitalists, emergency physicians, and anesthesiologists—are generally seen as "team players," but they still need to be induced to attend training. Inducement may simply take the form of a contract requirement or hourly reimbursement for training time, but the issue is a recurrent question and needs to be addressed.

A decade ago, as the first clinical systems were coming into common use, some hospitals paid physicians an amount that roughly accorded with their hourly rate of income. Not surprisingly, given the cost and growing adoption of such systems, this practice has become rare. Some hospitals simply make a demonstration of system competence a requirement for clinical privileges and leave it at that. The days when physicians angrily took their practice elsewhere are almost gone; whenever physicians threaten to take their patients to another local hospital, you can almost guarantee that the other hospital also has a clinical system in place—and a similar requirement.

Nonetheless, many hospitals still offer some inducement to physicians and—in many cases—nursing staff. The most common is continuing medical education (CME) credits, which are becoming a standard part of EHR training in North America, despite the paperwork and overhead involved. While many training sessions offer food, especially to physicians during evening classes, additional inducements—other than privileges and CME credits—are now uncommon.

COMMON TRAINING ISSUES

By now, training has become so universal that several common issues have been identified. These issues usually can be categorized under one of several themes: conflicting demands, inability to backfill clinical needs, failure of training technology, low retention of information, trainer burnout, insufficient number of trainers, and lack of management support.

Problem #1: Trainees Have Conflicting Clinical Duties

Solutions
- Ensure that clinical leaders understand that while they must provide adequate clinical coverage, training is both necessary and required.
- Enable flexible rescheduling to allow add-ins and make-up sessions.
- Ensure that syllabi include online learning and practice scenarios that do not need to be scheduled and can accommodate clinical surges.
- Ensure that registration and scheduling are both error free and real-time.
- Track no-shows, sick calls, and last-minute cancellations for follow-up.

Problem #2: Unexpected Needs for Clinical Coverage Occur While Trainees Are in Class

Solutions
- Anticipate that clinical surges will occur, and plan for them ahead of time.

- Maintain an active list of on-call staff.
- Ensure that upper management is aware of this problem and supports the solution.
- Use other available resources, such as part-time employees, pool employees, students, faculty, and traveling physicians (or *locum tenens*).
- Minimize or postpone other training requirements prior to go-live.
- Incorporate system training into routine training (e.g., new employee orientation time).

Problem #3: Training Technology Failure

Solutions
- Anticipate problems with system computers, user passwords, the practice domain, and the system catalog.
- Overestimate capacity and supply extra computers for backup.
- Make sure the IT department is on call during training.
- Freeze the build prior to training to prevent domain errors.
- If code changes are necessary, define and establish a change process.
- Use video tutorials (e.g., PowerPoint presentations, media files) if the live environment fails.
- Teach trainers and super-users to be troubleshooters.

Problem #4: Low Retention of Information Among Users

Solutions
- Ensure that training is clinical and role based.
- Offer refresher courses just prior to conversion.
- Offer a "play domain" in which users can practice.
- Communicate the need to practice new skills.
- Design job aids and make them available at conversion.

Problem #5: Burnout Among Trainers Working Long Hours and Teaching Repetitive Classes

Solutions
- Have a sufficient number of trainers and super-users and adequate backup support.
- Prevent combative or confrontational behavior by communicating expectations to trainees.
- Fully script the syllabi to reduce trainers' stress.
- Ensure there is sufficient IT support to guarantee a functioning domain.
- Oversee the trainers, recognize signs of stress, and intervene if necessary.
- Maintain good communication between the trainers and the rest of the individuals working on the project.

Problem #6: Too Few Trainers for Those Being Trained

Solutions
- Carefully predict the number of people to be trained and the number of trainers that will be required.
- Provide backup support and resources during training sessions.
- Use part-time trainers or part-time clinical personnel to provide flexibility.
- Temporarily reassign clinical or supervisory personnel as trainers.
- Hire a third-party firm to provide additional trainers.

Problem #7: Lack of Project Support for Training

Solutions
- Early in the project, solicit and obtain support from both the project management team and executive suite; ensure that they understand training resource needs (particularly clinical backfill), and market the training plan.

- Hold the project team responsible for training excellence as well as for other project deliverables.

KEY POINTS

- Communication
  - —is what they heard, not just what you said;
  - —must begin early, well before rumors begin;
  - —should be channeled through all available venues, including voice, phone, paper, meetings, and friends; and
  - —fails if you assume understanding and a shared context.
- Training
  - —begins on day one;
  - —also can be delivered in nonclassroom venues (e.g., department meetings);
  - —must be **clinical** and based on workflows (never train your staff to use a computer; train them to see patients);
  - —needs to be organized, scheduled, and assigned deadlines and a budget;
  - —needs to be structured by a clear set of syllabi tailored to privileges and workflow;
  - —must be sufficient and delivered as close to conversion as feasible; and
  - —can include "circling back" to optimize learning.

CHAPTER 8

Regulatory Issues

Agencies sometimes lose sight of common sense
as they create regulations.

—*Fred Thompson*

REGULATORY ISSUES ARE not new, but they are unprecedented as the driving force of medicine.

Like most technological change, regulatory change is generally unpredictable, but the institution of new—and often unexpected—regulatory requirements has become increasingly frequent over the past few decades. At the same time, the impact of these requirements has become increasingly pervasive, with significant implications for hospital finance and clinical workflow. There is little reason to suggest this trend will abate in the near future. In this chapter we look at regulatory compliance from a strategic perspective, bypassing details that are in flux or that pertain to nonhospital venues and focusing on the current issues and on how they may be mitigated or solved. We approach this discussion from the viewpoint of the executive suite rather than from the viewpoint of the individual tasked with the details of compliance or risk management, for the details not only change with time but also are addressed differently, sometimes significantly so, among hospitals.

As the pace of mandated regulatory compliance increases, hospitals are faced with three issues:

1. The unpredictability of regulations undercuts long-term hospital planning.

2. Regulatory compliance (and documentation) imposes a cost burden.
3. Physician compliance is often required but difficult to enforce.

These three factors make regulatory compliance onerous and demand advanced planning and careful budgeting. Balanced against these problems, several factors make compliance desirable.

First, the impetus behind regulations is often perceived as a desire to improve the quality and safety of patient care. It is difficult to argue with the intent, even if the regulation itself may be byzantine or occasionally counterproductive. In general, however, most regulations may be seen as benefitting patient care.

Second, hospitals can achieve significant financial gains by complying with regulations—at least initially. With regard to meaningful use, for example, Stage 1 is intended to help fund the otherwise unfunded mandate of EHR compliance. Unfortunately, such funding is not intended to be long term and is unlikely to cover the costs of compliance. Many hospitals view this funding source as "zero-sum" and benefiting only institutions that are ahead of the curve. Nonetheless, compliance does initially offer financial incentives.

Third, compliance is becoming increasingly required for hospital certification. Noncompliance can pose severe financial and licensing implications as well as legal risks for the hospital and its clinical staff. In this sense, compliance is the only way for the hospital to remain open.

REGULATION-FACING CARE?

Due to the increasing prevalence of regulation, hospitals commonly become "regulation facing" rather than "patient facing." In a simple, naïve sense, regulation-facing care is certainly undesirable and patient-facing care is much preferable, but a strictly business point of view argues that close attention to regulations is driven by considerations of risk management, financial planning, and legal concerns. However, a shift away from patient-facing care is not only a poor choice from the naïve perspective but also a risky one from a practical perspective: **Patient-facing care pays.**

Hospitals depend not only on finances and risk management but also on patient perceptions (e.g., Press Ganey scores) and the culture of their clinical staff. If the patient population perceives a hospital as caring for regulations to the exclusion of compassionate care, the hospital is as much at risk as it would be if it lost certification. Equally, the hospital needs a dedicated clinical staff—physicians, nurses, and allied professionals—to believe that patient care is the primary goal of the hospital. Any other perception will increase staff turnover, decrease recruitment, and prompt recurrent contractual wrangling and complaints. The long-term survival of a hospital depends on the perception that patient care is its cultural focus. **Patient care is primary; all regulatory compliance should be seen in this light.**

A useful distinction is that of primary and secondary goals of the hospital. The primary goal is patient care; secondary goals include financial gain, regulatory compliance, risk management, staff retention, and a host of other valid concerns. A hospital cannot survive without meeting most of its secondary goals, but the rationale for doing so is to meet the primary goal. Consider the example of Mother Teresa, who was famous for being a superb manager and fundraiser for her orphanage in India. She never went "into the red" or neglected the financial bottom line, but her rationale for meeting these **secondary** goals was to meet her **primary** philanthropic goal. Far from being naïve, this perspective simply reflects the reality of running a hospital. You must meet the bottom line so that you can deliver good patient care.

QUALITY: AN ELUSIVE GOAL

EHRs can be used to improve the quality of patient care, but having an EHR does not—by itself—improve medical care. Any change in the quality of care depends entirely on how the tool is used, and particularly on how you implement it. With attention to the design of the EHR, training, process changes, and other factors, patient care can reach a level of quality that it could never reach without the use of an EHR. Mere installation ensures nothing; innumerable risks and issues can arise when a hospital mistakenly believes that the EHR itself will provide value, independent of **how** it is used.

Fast delivery of care is desirable, but only in the context of solving the issues that brought the patient to the hospital and doing so in an effective and compassionate manner. Otherwise, patients may as well leave immediately after registration; they would thereby bring length of stay to zero. Decreasing length of stay is not a legitimate goal per se; it is only a convenient **marker** for the goal of improved patient care. There are many potentially misleading markers—for example, days in the hospital, readmission rates, and the need for repeat surgeries. These markers make an invaluable **contribution** to assessing the quality of patient care, but they do not measure quality in any direct sense and should never be confused with measures of quality per se.

Even markers that seem to measure important outcomes directly—for example, comparing hospitals on the basis of mortality or complication rates for a single diagnosis or surgical procedure—have no value without appropriate denominators. The best tertiary-care academic center might have twice the mortality of a small, community hospital, but if the community hospital treats only simple cases and refers all of its difficult cases to the academic center, the numbers may be misleading or simply wrong. If the tertiary-care hospital treats the cases that normally have ten times the mortality rate of those seen by the community hospital, we should be celebrating the fact that its superb care has lowered that mortality to **merely twice** that of the community hospital. In short, quality cannot—at least not simply and naïvely—be measured by any one number, whether that number be rate of mortality, cost, length of stay, complications, patient complaints, Press Ganey scores, an assessment of The Joint Commission, or a place in an annual survey of the best US hospitals. **Measuring quality requires finesse and sophistication.**

Assessment isn't the only problem. The pursuit of quality is prone to unexpected consequences. Any attempt to measure, let alone to improve, the quality of care can incur significant costs of its own. Assessment can degrade quality and produce meaningless results. Good intent is not enough: We must be sophisticated in our attempts to assess quality; look at the broad picture as we attempt to improve care; and, when we think we're done, check to see if we have succeeded or—to our shock—only made matters worse.

THE REGULATORY SPECTRUM

Current regulations can be divided into three categories: (1) regulations that address EHRs, (2) regulations that are largely independent of the form of the medical record, and (3) quasi-regulatory billing concerns. The first type of regulation requires hospitals to meet certain criteria to receive funding for an EHR, the second pertains to areas that can be improved via the use of an EHR, and the third—billing codes—is not actually a type of regulation. However, because billing codes have many of the same implications for workflow in hospitals, they often are addressed much as we would address any other regulation.

Meaningful Use

Part of the Health Information Technology for Economic and Clinical Health (HITECH) Act, *meaningful use* is a set of requirements issued by the Centers for Medicare & Medicaid Services (CMS). The intent of the act was to increase the quality and efficacy of healthcare, specifically through the use of EHRs and computer systems. Originally defined in the American Recovery and Reinvestment Act of 2009, meaningful use is meant to spur the use of a "certified EHR" for

- "meaningful" activities, such as e-prescribing;
- exchanging health information electronically; and
- reporting clinical quality and other measures.

Intent aside, a series of practical requirements was initially defined, along with stages, deadlines, and payment structures (see Exhibit 8.1 for details on Stage 1). The exact requirements for each stage have been altered since their original definition. Although there are separate requirements for hospitals and physicians (called "eligible professionals" [EPs] whether inpatient or outpatient), in this discussion we largely ignore the requirements for physicians and focus on hospital-based regulatory objectives.

Hospital objectives—inpatient requirements—are divided into two categories: (1) core objectives that all hospitals must meet and (2) menu objectives—a list of options from which hospitals can choose any five objectives. Originally, Stage 1 was to be in force by 2012, Stage 2 by 2013, and Stage 3 by 2015. Stage 2 has been pushed to 2014, and Stage 3 to 2016. The final requirements for Stage 2 were released in August 2012, while the requirements for Stage 3 remain in flux as this book goes to print. To meet the meaningful-use objectives successfully, hospitals will need to follow up on forthcoming changes and remain current with the latest CMS requirements.

In the next section, we discuss the predictable pitfalls hospitals may encounter in their efforts to achieve meaningful use as well as recommended strategies for overcoming them.

Practical Concerns

Although the details change, the overall strategy—and indeed the actual problems encountered in meeting the meaningful-use requirements—can be described to good effect. Most of the major issues faced by hospitals are generic and largely predictable. The

Exhibit 8.1: Meaningful-Use Stage 1 Hospital Requirements

Core Objectives (all required)	Measure
Demographics: sex, race, ethnicity, date of birth, language, and date and cause of death	These demographics are recorded as structured data in EHR for more than 50% of patients.
Vital signs, height, weight, blood pressure, body mass index, and growth charts (for children)	Height, weight, and blood pressure are recorded as structured data in EHR for more than 50% of patients aged 2 or older.
Up-to-date problem list of current and active diagnoses	At least one entry is recorded as structured data in EHR for more than 80% of patients.
Medication list	At least one entry is recorded as structured data in EHR for more than 80% of patients.
Allergy list	At least one entry is recorded as structured data in EHR for more than 80% of patients.
Smoking status (individuals aged 13 or older)	Smoking status is recorded as structured data in EHR for more than 50% of patients aged 13 or older.
Electronic copy of discharge instructions provided on request	Electronic copy of discharge instructions is provided to more than 50% of patients who request it.
Electronic copy of tests, problems, medications, allergies, discharge summary, and procedures provided on request	Electronic copy of this information is provided within three business days to more than 50% of patients who request it.

(Continued on next page)

Exhibit 8.1 (Continued)

Core Objectives (all required)	Measure
CPOE	At least one medication order is entered using CPOE for more than 30% of patients.
Drug–drug and drug–allergy checking	This functionality is enabled for the entire EHR reporting period.
Electronic exchange of clinical information among providers and "entities"	Perform at least one test of EHR's capacity to exchange clinical information electronically.
Clinical decision support rule: implement and track	At least one clinical decision support rule is implemented.
Protection of electronic health information	Analyze security risks, implement security updates, and correct security deficiencies.
Reporting of quality assurance measures to CMS or states	Successfully report clinical quality measures selected by CMS.

Menu Objectives (any five must be met)	Measure
Drug formulary checks	This functionality is enabled—and at least one formulary is accessible over the entire EHR reporting period.
Structured lab data	More than 40% of all lab results in positive/negative or numeric form are entered in EHR as structured data.
Generate lists of patients by conditions for quality assurance and other purposes	At least one report listing patients with a specific condition is generated.

Exhibit 8.1 (Continued)

Menu Objectives (any five must be met)	Measure
Use EHR to identify and provide patient-specific education	Patient-specific education resources are provided to more than 10% of patients.
Medication reconciliation	Medication reconciliation is done for more than 50% of patients transitioned to the hospital.
Summary of care when patient is transitioned/referred	A summary of care record is provided for more than 50% of patients transitioned/referred to another setting.
Submit electronic immunization data to registries	Perform at least one test of EHR's capacity to submit immunization data to registries electronically (unless none of the registries can receive data electronically).
Submit electronic syndrome surveillance data to public health agencies	Perform at least one test of EHR's capacity to submit syndrome surveillance data to agencies electronically (unless none of the agencies can receive data electronically).
Record advance directives for patients aged 65 or older	Advance directives are recorded as structured data in EHR for more than 50% of patients aged 65 or older.
Submit electronic lab data to public health agencies	Perform at least one test of EHR's capacity to submit lab data to agencies electronically (unless none of the agencies can receive data electronically).

Source: CMS (2012).

practical issues arising out of the hospital requirements for Stage 1 fall into several categories:

1. EHR certification per se is rarely an issue. All large, national vendors are certified; the only risk is posed by niche systems, which may be not only uncertified but also unable to pull and report the data necessary to meet the requirements for meaningful use (of any stage). Nevertheless, hospitals should review the certification of each vendor and—more important—the vendor's ability to meet the reporting requirements for meaningful use. Such checks are not only due diligence on the part of the hospital in choosing a vendor but also assurance of good-faith compliance on the part of the vendor in responding to future reporting needs. A reasonable contract requires the vendor to support adequate reporting, including future reporting requirements. When reporting requirements change, the vendor must be willing to stand behind the intent of the contract and assist in modifying its software to enable a hospital to meet those new requirements. Not surprisingly, the larger vendors are generally more able to accommodate unexpected changes, but even they may be unreliable when such needs arise. *Caveat emptor.*

2. The following requirements cause few or only trivial problems or changes:

   —The **allergy list** is central to medical care and causes few issues; it is a standard part of both medical culture and clinical workflow. In EHRs, however, there are slight but recurrent problems caused by the definition of an allergy (versus sensitivity, for example) or resulting from the unreliability of the patient's history. For example, nurses may incorrectly (or an EHR may force nurses to) document nausea caused by oral Augmentin as an allergy rather than as a sensitivity, thus triggering unnecessary allergy alerts to clinically indicated IV antibiotics.

Although this issue becomes more significant when an EHR is in routine use, it causes only minor difficulties during adoption and minimally disrupts efforts to meet the requirements of meaningful use.

—The requirement for an **exchange of information** among providers (or "entities") is not yet a practical issue because a simple demonstration suffices to meet the Stage 1 objective. This requirement will, however, go on to create future headaches (and costs) as it expands in subsequent stages to incorporate exchanging more complex data in various formats among health information exchanges and doing so reliably and routinely.

—The requirement for **security** is universal and not at all new; unfortunately, breaches are also universal (if uncommon) and are not new either. In general, this issue requires some additional thought to the management of security (e.g., passwords, portable data media, physician access to the EHR from outside the hospital), but at least in principle it is well understood. Specifics have been added to this requirement, including access control (e.g., passwords), emergency access, automatic logoff (although idle time until logoff has not been specified), audit log, integrity (e.g., maintaining messages, verifying lack of alteration, detecting alteration of audits), authentication (of users), general encryption, and encryption during exchange of information.

—The requirement for **drug formulary checks** (see Chapter 4) is incumbent on any conversion, and meaningful use adds no significant burden in this regard.

—**Digital laboratory data** are—like the drug formulary— part and parcel of having an EHR, and no additional work is necessary to meet the meaningful-use requirement.

3. The following requirements involve modification of policy, workflow, or both but seldom create lasting issues for either clinical adoption or enforcement:

—Additional **demographic data** must be obtained. Concerns have been expressed regarding the clinical (as opposed to legal or financial) value of some parts of this data set, but the requirement is relatively easy to meet and has caused few or no adoption issues among hospital staffs.

—Additional **vital signs and similar data** must be obtained. Some venues, such as EDs, have pointed out that height rarely plays a role in clinical decision making regarding adults. The requirement remains, however, and most such venues have (with grumbling) simply gone along with the requirement, understanding its value for the pediatric, oncologic, and other settings.

—**Smoking history** must be obtained. The information required is more detailed than the smoking-related data that have historically been documented in medicine, and initial regulatory demands have been contradictory with regard to the age requirement and other parameters. In practice, however, the major issue is simply getting the staff used to obtaining the required details and documenting the data.

—Sending patients home with an **electronic copy of their discharge instructions** and information regarding their diagnoses, medications, procedures, and so forth has caused initial problems for many hospitals, although the "patient portal," which provides patients password-protected access to their personal data, is becoming the common solution. The requirement causes minor practical and planning difficulties but poses few difficulties for adoption and enforcement among clinical staff.

—The requirement for at least **one clinical decision support (CDS) rule** is easy to meet, although the issue becomes more troublesome as multiple rules are added to the system, causing alert fatigue and clarifying the need to carefully tailor clinical rules to appropriate and effective use. With regard to CDS, more is clearly not better.

—The requirement to **gather and submit quality assurance data** appears simple, but some complexity becomes apparent upon examining the details. From the options available to meet this requirement, hospitals must choose a quality measure it can obtain without undue effort or cost, not necessarily one that is useful. Prior to the use of the EHR, expensive human resources had to manually extract and compile these data; with the EHR, this task is potentially easier, but it can be difficult to ensure that the data are both valid and reliable. A surprising amount of thought is required to precisely define a rule that will pull meaningful data, and even then the resulting data may not fulfill essential parts of the intended goal. With logical planning and forethought, however, meeting this requirement is not a significant issue.

—Generating a **list of patients with a specific condition** is—*prima facie*—easy; however, ease in this case depends on maintaining an accurate list of diagnoses (see category #4 later in this section) and on the vendor's ability to generate reports based on these data. The former depends on careful definition of the clinical workflow and on the rate of EHR adoption among physicians and nurses; the latter is addressed by careful vendor selection (see category #1 earlier in this section). With these two caveats, generating such a list is seldom a problem.

—Generating **patient-specific education** is a typical function of most EHRs (or can be added as a subscription), and the impact is negligible, save for the requirement that the information be not only generated but actually provided to the patient. The latter action requires that nurses (and occasionally physicians) ensure that the patient receives the information. Set at more than 10 percent during Stages 1 and 2, the proportion of patients to whom this information must be provided may climb in Stage 3.

—**Immunization registries** vary around the country, notably between states as well as occasionally within states, which has made it difficult to meet their differing requirements. The situation is improving rapidly, however. More and more registries are accepting electronic immunization data in common (rather than idiosyncratic) formats, and vendors are becoming increasingly adept at designing their systems to provide this information. The same is true of other types of national medical registries, such as for trauma, domestic abuse, child abuse, animal bites, and other reportable legal and epidemiologic data.

—Means of acquiring **syndrome surveillance data** have lagged in terms of sophistication, but submission of these data is (like immunization data) seldom a problem for health departments that are capable of accepting them electronically. While some health departments are still clinging hopelessly to paper, others have simply adopted byzantine forms of their previous paper interfaces and put these forms on a website. The most advanced (and appropriately funded) health departments, however, accept coded data easily.

—**Advance directives** are seldom a practical problem, but two issues arise repeatedly in most hospitals. The first occurs in obtaining a decision from patients and families, in that there is frequently reluctance on the part of either clinicians or patients (and family members) to discuss and finalize advance directives, although this issue is certainly not a new one. The second issue is where to place such information in the EHR. Some hospitals place it front and center—for example, on the banner bar or on a tracking view where it is readily visible to clinicians and easily found when a code occurs. Other hospitals, concerned that the information be kept strictly confidential, have made it harder to find, often necessitating multiple clicks or even an additional password. While this placement respects the need for patient confidentiality, it wreaks havoc during codes when immediate clinical decisions need to be made. It may take a minute or more to find the advance directive (let alone interpret it, unless it is concise and clearly phrased) when the physician may have only seconds to decide whether to intubate, shock, or start CPR. Even patients who strongly prefer not to receive resuscitation often are given resuscitative measures because the clinical staff can't locate the advance directive in time. Placement of advance directives is an example of a situation in which opposing risks need to be balanced to optimize care.

—The submission of **lab data to public health agencies**—like the problem with registries and syndrome surveillance— depends on the ability of the health agency to receive the data more than it depends on the ability of the hospital to submit it. Typically, the only concern from the hospital's viewpoint is that it maintain confidentiality to the extent permitted by law and that it adequately "shake hands" with the system used by the public health agency.

4. The following requirements involve workflow changes and may create substantial obstacles to adoption by clinical staff:

—An up-to-date, accurate **list of diagnoses** must be obtained, which always raises the issue of who (nurse or physician) documents and maintains this information as well as how this information is handled within the physician's workflow. Typically, physicians want to "own" the diagnoses list, yet they also want nurses to enter the majority of the information for them. The caveat "when everyone is responsible, no one is responsible" applies to all cases of shared responsibility. Most hospitals finally come to the decision that—as part of hospital privileges— physicians are responsible for the accuracy of the diagnoses list, and the hospital enforces this directive through quality assurance and the medical executive committee.

—The **medication list** causes a surprising amount of angst, despite the fact that such lists are not new. The problem is many-headed: (1) It is harder for the nurse to enter the medications into a computer than it was to write them down on paper (slowing both nurses' and physicians' workflow); (2) the physicians must have an accurate, immediate, real-time list of medications at the time of admission to do a medication reconciliation (intensifying the ill will they have for the nurses who haven't yet finished obtaining this list); and (3) there is still a moderate degree of mismatch in available formularies, making both entry and reconciliation of medications more frustrating than they were in the paper world. The result is almost universal difficulties with this workflow and predictable problems with adoption. The usual solutions are to devote more resources to achieving formulary matches, adjust the nursing workflow in the ED and during admissions, and train physicians on medication reconciliation and enforce it (see discussion on this issue later in this list).

—**CPOE** itself has become less and less of an issue over the past few years due to both the growing physician acceptance of an emerging medical standard and the improvements that have been made to the system interfaces used to place orders. Nonetheless, CPOE remains the single most easily defined and universally shared issue in physician EHR adoption and depends heavily on the interface, the catalog, and various other factors (such as order set design, which was addressed in previous chapters). Due care must be exercised in defining the CPOE percentage because both the numerator (number of orders entered by the physician) and the denominator (total number of orders entered) can be surprisingly difficult to pin down precisely, and hospitals that have an inaccurate definition may fail to meet CPOE requirements (to read about the experience of a community hospital in Florida, see the box on the following page).

—**Interaction checking** is technically fairly easy but causes considerable problems, almost exclusively due to "alert fatigue." The general response has been to minimize the number of triggers and tailor the interaction alerts seen by the physician or nurse while showing the gamut of alerts to the pharmacy staff. The key question in defining a useful alert is not "Is there a potential drug interaction?" but rather "Is this alert likely to cause the physician to change the order?" Unimportant alerts, or alerts that rarely alter physician decisions, cause poor patient care and increase patient risk. Every trivial alert makes it harder to recognize a critical alert.

—**Medication reconciliation** is almost a universal issue for physicians. As noted previously, it is partly due to issues with the accuracy of the medication list itself, partly due to the inability to obtain automatic drug matches from internal and external formularies, and partly due to

---

Poorly Defined Numerators Equal Poor Compliance

A large community hospital on the west coast of Florida had instituted CPOE with what should have been success, given that the physicians reported that they were indeed placing most of their orders through the computer. However, the monthly statistics showed that CPOE was well below the 30 percent Stage 1 requirement, without apparent cause. The system had a form of order set that could be placed into a "planned" state by the physician and then initiated by the nurse. While the physician had plainly entered the orders as CPOE, the system was recording the orders as verbal rather than CPOE because the nurses had been the ones initiating the orders. The definition of the numerator was altered to reflect the physician entry of the planned order sets, and CPOE was immediately shown to be well above 70 percent.

---

problems with clunky interfaces, which cause delays in the physician workflow. The majority of physicians complain about the unnecessary difficulties inherent in medication reconciliation.

There also are hidden pitfalls in a number of the requirements. Just because you have gathered data doesn't mean that the data are valid or reliable. As in the example about planned versus initiated orders counting as CPOE (see the box on the previous page), definitions can play havoc with data. In the case of CPOE, another issue is that of triage orders in the emergency setting. These orders have been predefined by the physicians, initiated by the nurses, and signed by the physician who is caring for the patient. Do

---

Inadequate Formulary Matching Hampers Compliance

Medication reconciliation (meds rec) is a recurrent problem. In many systems, the initial obstacle has taken the following form: The physician is reviewing the list of medications that the patient takes at home. On the list is a perfectly common oral medication that the nurse has (appropriately) entered as "furosemide 40 mg po qd." Yet when the physician tries to perform an admission meds rec, there is no automatic match in the hospital formulary and the physician is forced to reenter precisely the same information as an inpatient medication order rather than have the system find "furosemide 40 mg po qd" as an orderable. Although the difficulties lie in matching formularies, the physician's conclusion is that the system doesn't work. Once the matching formularies have been set up, medication matches are routinely made more than 70 percent of the time. To get physicians to use the system, you should ensure matches well exceed 90 percent.

---

such orders constitute CPOE? Similar questions arise with regard to defining standing or protocol orders, such as insulin protocols, venous thromboembolism prophylaxis, and other orders that prompt "routine" nursing responses.

The same definition problems are present in attempts to meet regulatory guidelines other than those of meaningful use. In defining adherence to the guidelines for antibiotic administration to patients admitted for pneumonia, many hospitals find themselves playing with the definition of when the patient was admitted, diagnosed, or seen by a physician. While such adjustments are understandable given the costs of noncompliance and the linguistic fuzziness of certain regulations, three caveats must be kept in mind when defining how the system should view and retrieve data for reporting:

1. **Inaccurate data:** Reported data are only as good as the data that have been entered in the system. The most common problem (but only one among dozens) is the definition of when the patient is seen by the physician (e.g., the door-to-doctor time). Physicians may "claim" a patient long before they actually see the patient, or they may get involved in a medical crisis and care for a patient for a long time before they actually document that they are seeing the patient. These errors can occur intentionally (claiming patients to increase income) or unintentionally (claiming patients and then getting involved in a code), but the outcome is the same: Unreliable data become the basis for reporting.

2. **Inaccurate reports:** If the entered data are inaccurate (e.g., as a result of human error) or if the definition of the report is flawed (e.g., the numerator or denominator for determining the percentage of CPOE orders placed is poorly defined), the reported figures not only will be incorrect but also can lead to costly decisions. Whether an abnormal report suggests a problem that isn't real or a normal report hides a critical issue, the hospital risks resources, finances, and regulatory

consequences that could be prevented by careful reporting definitions.

3. **Regulatory risks:** Regulators may not agree with your data or your conclusions. Flawed data and flawed reports run the risk of appearing intentional, particularly if they are inaccurately optimistic. The risks of having inaccurate data and generating inaccurate reports are not simply internal but can involve external sanctions and costs.

Meeting Standards

There is a general, global movement toward increasing the quality of patient care. It has been accompanied—and enforced—by an increasing emphasis on regulatory standards in the United States and elsewhere. Such standards include—but are not limited to—meaningful use. For example, The Joint Commission and CMS have promulgated a set of eight core measures that is in most ways independent of the implementation of EHR systems. The

---

Current Reportable Measures from CMS and The Joint Commission

AMI (Acute Myocardial Infarction)

HF (Heart Failure)

PNE (Pneumonia)

SCIP (Surgical Care Improvement Project)

PR (Pregnancy and Related Conditions)

CAC (Children's Asthma Care)

VTE (Venous Thromboembolism)

STK (Stroke)

---

advent of EHRs has made it easier to document compliance but has demanded greater attention to definition of the reports (e.g., numerators and denominators) and to the accuracy of the data gathered. No longer can hospitals rely on the expensive expertise of staff members who can sift through paper records and collate extracted data. The task has shifted from those who gather the data to those who have the expertise to **define how the system should gather** the data.

Each of the eight measures has a number of defined data elements, which may be intuitively clear to those extracting the data but remarkably difficult to pin down in a computer reporting system without making unintentional errors. For a simple example, the first data element required for the acute myocardial infarction (AMI) measure is "aspirin at arrival," which can be fulfilled by documenting that the patient took an aspirin prior to arrival, that the patient has an aspirin allergy, or that the patient refused to take the aspirin. While these exceptions are clear to human reviewers, pinpointing the correct set of locations where these exceptions reside can be remarkably difficult, as it may require the computer to look in several places for many possible forms of documentation.

This same practical difficulty pertains to reporting systems that are intended to be used to search for smoking cessation advice (for the heart failure [HF] and pneumonia [PNE] measures), discontinuation of antibiotics (for the Surgical Care Improvement Project [SCIP] measure), and the various possible forms of—and exceptions to—appropriate venous thromboembolism (VTE) prophylaxis. These data elements appear eminently clear and obvious until we attempt to point the computer to a single, unambiguous location for retrieval of the data in question. In short, computer reporting for regulatory requirements calls for a keen intelligence and an appreciation for both the complexities and ambiguities of real-life clinical care and the way in which data are stored and located in a system.

KEY POINTS

- Quality drives regulation but has other implications:
  —The goal of regulation is better patient care.
  —Patient-facing care pays long-term dividends.
  —Regulation-facing care can incur long-term costs.
- Meaningful use is the most common current concern:
  —The requirements change with each successive stage.
  —Most hospitals can meet the requirements.
  —Predictable issues can often be addressed or avoided.
- Reporting from data requires careful planning:
  —Minimize **inaccurate data** entry and documentation.
  —Be wary of **poor definitions** of data elements.
  —Compare final reporting with expectations and perceptions.

CHAPTER 9

Devices, Technology, and Infrastructure

*Any sufficiently advanced technology
is indistinguishable from magic.*

—*Arthur C. Clarke*

DEVICES THAT UNDERLIE the clinical use of EHRs are continually changing. When evaluating project needs—such as for an implementation—we must make reasonably accurate predictions about what devices will be available, what capabilities these devices will offer, and what users will actually use in clinical practice over a time frame of 6 to 12 months. Many devices are expensive to purchase and expensive to replace, making it desirable to ensure that the ones we purchase will still be useful over the next few years.

Technical changes are more amenable to prediction than are the corresponding social changes (e.g., new regulatory requirements, state and federal laws, payment structures) that invoke them. We foresaw the iPad several years ago, as well as its clinical pattern of use and its limitations. Other devices and technologies are also predictable and will soon enter routine clinical use.

In this chapter, we review the uses and pitfalls of current devices, as well as explore the current "technology vector," to give you a handle on where best (and not) to invest when budgeting for tomorrow's hospital infrastructure. We focus almost exclusively on the devices used daily by clinical personnel in delivering patient care (e.g., devices used by physicians and nurses on the wards) and slight other devices that are not part of the day-to-day use of the EHR.

GENERAL STRATEGY

More and more hospitals are becoming remote hosted organizations (RHOs) that rely on vendors to manage their hardware, software, and clinical information storage and retrieval. Although this approach is costly, it is often cost-effective, considering initial system prices, updates, reliability, and maintenance staff. Single vendors can often manage these issues—and their associated costs—more efficiently than can the individual hospital. While the RHO strategy is far from universal, there is a clear trend in that direction and no obvious reason why it should stop short of complete saturation of the market. Current conditions suggest that—within the next decade—almost all hospitals will be adopting an RHO strategy, except perhaps the largest national hospital chains. Conditions may change, but the trend is clear.

The focus of this chapter, however, is on devices rather than systems. While the current trend is for systems to be managed by single vendors (the RHO model), desktops and portable systems are an altogether different matter. In the case of desktops and similar units, the hospital generally budgets for and owns them; in the case of portable devices, such as smartphones and iPads, there is a clear trend toward purchase and ownership by users rather than by the hospital (i.e., BYOD, or "bring your own device").

Desktop units continue to offer improved capabilities, but the role of the desktop as an element of clinical workflow has been relatively stable. Users tend to access the desktop in a central location, sit down alone, and interact with the system in a single, prolonged session. Even in the emergency and ICU settings, users often access multiple patient records and make multiple medical decisions during a single session. Essentially, the only changes in desktop workflow have been larger screens (essential for radiology images and ICU care) and voice recognition. Most of the other technical improvements have been incremental and have had minimal impact on the pattern of clinical workflow.

Compared to desktops, or even laptops, the current generation of portable devices—as exemplified by the iPad—is markedly different with regard to function and clinical workflow. The current tablet-type device has created a clinical workflow that was not previously present, although the most portable of laptops (e.g., those designed by Motion Computing and Toughbook) had begun to move in this direction. Curiously, this workflow somewhat echoes the old workflow staff used when carrying paper charts, especially during morning rounds. Users access the tablet as they see patients and usually don't sit down to use the device; they may take the device from ward to ward and floor to floor in the hospital (wireless infrastructure permitting). The tablet is small enough to be carried easily; some hospitals even offer their staff the option of adding pockets specifically made for these devices to their lab coats.

A key feature of the tablet-type device is its plethora of other (e.g., recreational) applications that encourage personal and home use, which was not typical of previous devices. The result has been a wholesale shift in the pattern of ownership: Physicians now desire access to the EHR via their personal devices rather than via a hospital-supplied device. Most hospitals allow (or even encourage) the use of personal devices—generally tablets and smartphones. This trend has an upside—it doesn't cost the hospital anything if the user buys the device—and a downside—it requires careful attention to security and confidentiality concerns. Hospitals usually have several ground rules pertaining to the use of personal devices:

- The user owns the device and is responsible for any repair or replacement.
- The hospital will help the user access the EHR but does not offer other support.

- The user must adhere to normal confidentiality and password agreements.
- The device must not store patient information.

A few hospitals have gone further and required that the user activate the optional device login and password (as well as the EHR login and password) and a timed logoff. While hospitals that own such devices may activate the option to remotely wipe information from them, no hospital has yet required that it be able to remotely wipe user-owned devices. Such a requirement would be unlikely to survive staff backlash if a hospital were to do so.

In summary, **we recommend that users be allowed to own their devices; security can be maintained with forethought and planning**.

The trend toward personal ownership notwithstanding, many hospitals still choose to purchase portable devices, whether laptops or tablets. When purchasing portable devices, hospitals need to consider several parameters, many of which equally apply to the purchase of desktop devices:

- Ease of cleaning (especially keyboards, which are difficult to sterilize)
- Weight (and how easy it is to carry [e.g., type of handles])
- Screen size (especially for radiology views)
- Docking (e.g., for a second keyboard or screen and for charging)
- Ability to take clinical photos (and upload them to the EHR)
- Ability to scan (especially ID bands, drugs, and pumps)
- Voice recognition (fidelity, speed, and location of user files)
- Durability (e.g., if dropped from gurney height)
- Cost (and cost of accessories [e.g., special type of stylus], repairs, and support)
- Theft protection (and whether it can be located or wiped of data)
- Ease of signing in (Is login delayed?)

- Ease of battery swap (Can it be hot-swapped?)
- Battery life (actual, not the manufacturer's claim)
- Keyboard ease of use
- Touchscreen (or multi-touch capability)

The gamut of computer devices includes desktops, drop-down units (which unfold from the wall outside of patient rooms), computers/workstations on wheels (often called COWs and WOWs), tablets, smartphones, handheld devices (including scanners), and pocket PCs. In addition, many hospitals now employ specialized phones (e.g., Vocera) that enable hands-free communication, patient tracking devices, and "smart rooms" (in which computers are installed in beds, walls, and doors). These devices, their capabilities, and their interfaces change rapidly and quickly

---

Don't Trust, but Verify

One manufacturer claimed that its lightweight tablet could stand up to 10 Gs and wouldn't be damaged in clinical use even if it were dropped. During the demonstration, one physician asked about typical events, such as dropping the tablet from a patient gurney onto a hard floor surface. The salesman replied, "It's guaranteed not to damage our tablet. It won't even stop working. It's fully protected!" The physician lifted the tablet to waist level, held it out by one finger over the concrete floor, and asked, "Then you won't mind if I try it?"

The salesman gasped and clutched at the tablet desperately to prevent it from falling to the floor. Looking embarrassed, he contended, "Well, it *probably* won't damage it."

Vendor claims may be accurate, but they are, after all, only claims.

---

become antiquated. The cost and effort of maintaining them have instigated two trends: the use of devices with multiple capabilities and a preference for buying all of a hospital's devices from a single manufacturer. The same trend is evident with purely clinical devices, such as picture archiving and communication systems (PACS) and EKG machines.

WIRELESS INFRASTRUCTURE

Most modern devices, whether essentially a computer or essentially clinical in nature, rely on wireless communication. Particularly in older hospitals, the wireless infrastructure can be limiting in that it may prevent the use of devices that are becoming common in clinical care. Even in modern buildings, the wireless infrastructure can create havoc at times.

For implementing CPOE or accessing routine clinical data, the limitations of the wireless system are seldom evident. These limitations do, however, become problematic (causing frustration and slowing patient care) in two common contexts:

1. Transmission of high-bandwidth data, such as large radiology files
2. Templated documents and voice recognition, which require high-speed responses

While radiology files (especially CT and MRI files with multiple views and dynamic data interpretation, as opposed to static files) are infamous for requiring high bandwidth, the problem of templated documents is often overlooked. At issue is the response time: The user clicks and then—after a short delay—the interface responds to the click. In a wired system, the delay is essentially imperceptible, but the response can be markedly delayed in a wireless system. CPOE users often ignore the delay and "lead" the system by clicking ahead. For example, they click an order, sign the order, and refresh the screen by clicking the appropriate areas of the screen before the computer responds to their first click. Users ignore the delay, even when it is perceptible, because they can accurately predict the response of the computer.

Templated documentation, however, is a different matter, and it becomes difficult for users to tolerate a delay. Templates usually are based on a modal entry system in which the first click documents a positive finding, the second click documents a negative finding, and the third click leaves the finding blank again. If users click once and nothing happens, they are often unsure whether the system registered the click. They often pause and then click a

---

Use a Stopwatch: How Slow Is Slow?

The intensivists in a large hospital in Iowa noted that it was difficult to access patient X-rays during ICU rounds. The attending physicians and residents normally "toured" the ICU with two computers on wheels—one for viewing data and the other for placing orders—with one resident assigned to each computer. The physicians complained that it was taking too long to bring up X-rays, yet technical support assured them that the wireless signal was good throughout the ICU.

Taking a stopwatch and timing 16 consecutive patients, I found that the average loading time for a simple chest X-ray (not including CTs or MRIs with windows or multiple views) was 2 minutes and 20 seconds. The problem was not the signal but the software used to access the images. The CMIO hadn't been impressed by the common complaint of "slowness" but was quick to address the issue when these data were presented to him.

—Michael Fossel

---

second time to obtain a response (and may repeat this same process several times). When the system finally catches up with users' clicks, in many cases the resulting documentation does not reflect users' intent, causing frustration and forcing them to redo the documentation. While most users tolerate a small delay when entering orders, it is maddening during documentation.

Moreover, wireless signal strength alone is no guarantee. Signal reflections can occur, multiple users can fill the available bandwidth, or the system can be busy with background tasks. For whatever reason, the only way to ensure that the wireless system will adequately support templated documentation is to stress the system with multiple users in actual clinical use. From the clinical perspective—particularly for documentation—the wireless system must be reliable and have a large bandwidth, and its response time must be imperceptible. Certain physicians—notably hospitalists—also require a wireless system that allows them to migrate between floors and between wards without losing connectivity from their portable devices; loss of connectivity forces them to log on repeatedly, thus slowing workflow. Good clinical practice demands a wireless connection that

- is broad and fast, without perceptible delay;
- is tested by actual clinical use rather than by signal meters;
- can maintain connection between floors and wards;
- does not degrade into "dead spots" in clinical areas; and
- can support multiple users during peak rounding times.

DATA DISPLAY

There is almost no such thing as a computer that is too fast or a screen that is too large. The latter—a large screen—is universally in demand but particularly so in the ICU, for any tracking board, and for viewing radiology results. Many users also demand high resolutions (a large number of pixels), but the limits of human optical resolution and the requirement for massive amounts of clinical data combine to push for larger screens, regardless of resolution. The current norm, often considered the minimum size for clinical use, is a high-resolution screen that is greater than 20 inches diagonally.

If a screen is placed in patient rooms, it should not face the patient. While this placement allows the patient to view the data, it also ensures that the nurse will have her back to the patient, undermining the nurse–patient relationship and the patient's perception of compassionate care. Nurses—and physicians for that matter—should be patient facing rather than computer facing, wherever feasible, and the environment should support this behavior.

ASSESSING DEVICES

Devices change so rapidly that the rule of thumb is to assess and budget for them early in the project but purchase (or lease) them at the last feasible moment. As noted earlier, any device must be evaluated with regard to a number of parameters, the two most important (and often conflicting) parameters being ease of clinical use and cost. While much of the assessment can be done by the IT department using available data, clinical assessment—equally necessary—is more difficult. To some extent, clinical assessment can be based on published rankings and usage statistics from similar hospitals with similar clinical environments. Ultimately, however, the devices must be assessed by the clinical personnel who actually will be using them.

While devices are usually assessed in-house during "device fairs," several caveats must be kept in mind:

- Physicians and nurses who attend device fairs are seldom representative of clinical staff.
- Opinions expressed in a device fair may not bear out in clinical use.

- After actually using a device, clinical staff almost invariably choose a different one.

Caveats notwithstanding, there are two clear benefits to holding a device fair. The first is that the users can handle and use the devices and thereby are able to rule out some devices and strongly reconsider others. This reevaluation is fine if based on practical comments, such as "I don't see how we could possibly clean this device" or "I didn't realize this device would be so heavy." Fanciful or emotional comments, such as "I like the look of this device" or "I hate the company that makes that device" might conceivably be useful but should be taken with a grain of salt. Specific points that have an impact on clinical use should be noted and used in the assessment. Any reasonable clinical user will have a better idea of what will work than will an IT specialist who doesn't have clinical duties. The second value of a device fair is ensuring the perception that clinical users were consulted and that their opinions—as professionals—make a difference. Clearly, many nonclinical issues—cost comes to mind immediately—must play a role in the decision to purchase a device, but clinical utility is of equal importance, and clinical users need to perceive that it matters.

There are almost always significant benefits to purchasing all devices from a single vendor, including cost breaks, ease of servicing the hardware, and simpler internal device support. On the other hand, (1) it is difficult to find a single vendor who can supply the entire spectrum of devices a hospital needs; (2) even when one vendor can supply devices for multiple uses and multiple settings, the best vendor for one clinical setting is not always the best (or even an adequate) vendor for another clinical setting; and (3) all users are different, each tending to favor a different device, even within a single clinical setting. Most hospitals compromise on the single versus multiple vendor question, using one major vendor and a few secondary vendors as necessary to balance these three factors. Cost and maintenance remain an important consideration, but clinical utility and user preference are equally important.

A large-volume ED went live with CPOE and purchased two-dozen state-of-the-art laptops, basing its selection on evaluations by administration and the IT department. The ED physicians were encouraged to use the new laptops—which they all did, for at least the first two weeks—but within a month, the physicians had stopped using the laptops altogether. They uniformly stated that it was easier to see the patient and return to their desktop computers than to carry the laptops and log on a second time when they sat at the desktops.

The hospital had purchased rather than leased the new laptops, and the CFO was relieved when they were finally resold at a loss.

No matter how clear the final decision appears, never commit to a device until you must. Devices invariably improve, and prices may even drop, often just after the contract has been signed. In addition, avoid capital purchases for devices that the clinical users, particularly the physicians, may later reject. Some hospitals carefully consider leasing devices until they are convinced that their physicians and nurses will actually use them.

Rule one: Assess early, purchase late.
Rule two: Lease now, purchase later.

THE TECHNOLOGY CURVE

Any technology—whether cars, audio equipment, refrigerators, or computers—follows a curve that describes its features and complexity. In general, devices start out with few features (but are easy to use), then gain features (but become hard to use), and then finally mature, offering even more features (but become easy to use again). The technology itself precedes its ease of use.

Most technology markets are initially driven by function; only when a technology matures do considerations of human factors and ease of use become the drivers. Consider audio technology as an example (although we could equally look at telephones, televisions, or automobiles): The first home record players were simple to use but offered few features and performed poorly. As audio technology matured, hi-fi systems became complex and confusing to most home users but offered more features and performed better. Today, personal audio devices (e.g., the iPod) are mindlessly simple to use, but they have a wealth of features and their performance is excellent.

Current generations of electronic health systems are much the same as any technology and follow the same curve of features and ease of use. Although EHRs have offered progressively better features and performance, they are still notoriously hard to use and require clinical users to complete numerous hours of training. The current generation of EHRs is the first to become more user-friendly, feature better-designed clinical interfaces, and require users to complete fewer hours of training.

The hallmark of a well-designed technology is that it requires little training: The better the design, the less training required. Current EHRs need to be improved a great deal more before clinical training is itself sufficient and little or no EHR-specific training is necessary for the seasoned clinician. Even now, however, we are seeing improvements, including the advent of natural language processing, voice recognition, and clinical decision support engines. A well-designed EHR requires clinical education, not device education.

FUTURE DEVICES

Many functions that echo the past are on the horizon. Vendors are struggling to enable systems to recognize, analyze, and act on verbal orders. Systems taking verbal orders will—much as the secretary or nurse once did—question the use of medications in the face of allergies or interactions, offer alternative therapies, and request additional information. Not only are vendors moving in this direction; rudimentary, commercial combinations of voice recognition and simple artificial intelligence, such as the technology that drives Siri in the current iPhone, are already available.

Future iterations will incorporate clinical decision support, striving to increase patient safety while decreasing costs. Moreover, such systems will be able to move billing, data documentation, and reporting considerations into the background, removing such artificial structures as the current ICD (and other billing-oriented) diagnostic codes and allowing the clinical user to focus on clinical interventions. Whatever the precise details of future systems, we will have the technical ability to bring back an emphasis on

---

A Real-World Example of a Device Strategy

A large, academic institution in the South converted its clinics to CPOE and electronic documentation. When asked to describe its experience and device strategy in the ambulatory setting, it gave the following response:

> Our devices vary between clinics. We set up a simulation clinic using various devices and then had the physicians and their staffs come through to test their workflow and to evaluate device options. It was much like the device fair that we used for our inpatient conversion. We gave each clinic a budgeted price so it could choose its own devices as it saw fit, but each clinic could also choose to go higher as long as it paid the difference. Most use thin clients in physician offices, nursing stations, and some hallway work areas. One clinic uses wall-mounted fold-down devices. Many have computers in their exam rooms.

---

clinical thinking and improve decision making while handling nonclinical tasks without wasting clinical personnel.

The coming transition to voice recognition, artificial intelligence, and clinical decision support as the basis for good clinical care is the most obvious and substantial change on the horizon, but not the only one. Current computer systems—none in current use in the modern hospital—are capable of recognizing individuals. This capability could be used not only to identify users (as a method of logging on to the EHR) but also to recognize and register patients as well as ensure that the right patient is given the right medication. Individuals can also be identified using voice, fingerprints, retina prints, iris patterns, and even typing patterns (a user's unique pattern of clicking, scrolling, and typing).

Although the future of medicine is usually discussed in terms of medications, robot surgery, advanced imaging, telomeres, and even nanotechnology, much of our medical future will be shaped by EHRs and the devices we employ. Current devices—and the software that we run on them—still have a long way to go in terms of both ease of use and support of good patient care.

KEY POINTS

- Selection of all devices, whether stationary or portable, involves a compromise between
    —the cost of the device and its maintenance, and
    —its clinical functions and ease of use.
- Many hospitals are moving toward physician-owned portable devices because
    —it is cheaper for the hospital and easier to keep up with new technology,
    —users have the technology they find preferable and optimal for care, and
    —the security and confidentiality of most personal devices can be managed.

- Wireless systems can be limiting due to
  —insufficient bandwidth to handle a large number of users;
  —insufficient bandwidth to handle large radiology files;
  —insufficient speed to process templated electronic documentation; and
  —dead spots, especially between floors and units.
- Large or multiple screens are required for
  —ICUs and similar settings; and
  —easy, simultaneous access to PACS and EHR data.
- When assessing devices
  —hold a device fair and clarify clinical staff's needs and desires,
  —don't purchase until necessary, and
  —consider leasing first.

CHAPTER 10

Implementation

'Tis not enough to help the feeble up,
but to support them after.

—William Shakespeare

UNTIL THE PAST few years, implementation was the central focus of most EHR projects for two reasons: (1) It was the event that defined the deadlines and requirements for the project, and (2) the major issues of both patient care and clinical adoption came to a head during this event. Currently, most hospitals have at least a partial EHR and—as a result—the emphasis is shifting to the addition of new EHR functions and the optimization of functions already in place. Nonetheless, the implementation, culminating in the conversion (go-live), is still the most significant event and the defining goal of most projects.

The previous chapters in this book have dealt with governance, education, and other aspects of EHR projects. These and similar topics are not repeated in this chapter, but they may be looked at afresh in the context of the conversion event rather than in the context of the project as a whole. The majority of this chapter focuses on the practical issues—such as staffing, issue tracking, and support—that arise during a conversion.

THE IMPORTANCE OF THE CONVERSION

The significance of the conversion cannot be overestimated, for it is with the conversion in mind that we have made the major clinical decisions; designed the daily clinical tools; and set the policies that will have a direct impact on physicians, nurses, and other clinical personnel as they deliver patient care. Correctly handled, the transition to an electronic hospital will be smooth; incorrectly handled, it will bring about recriminations, grudging compliance, and resentment among clinical staff. Moreover, it is during conversion that we see its actual impact on regulatory compliance, patient safety, and financial success.

For an analogy, imagine we are building a new hospital. Prior to reading this chapter, we would have designed the facility, finalized the blueprints, and signed the contract. The structure is going up, we are in the final phases of installing equipment and hiring staff, and we are preparing to admit our first patients. In this chapter, we outline and discuss how to ensure success as we open the new facility for patient care. There are myriad strategic decisions still to make and policies to set into motion carefully and correctly. These decisions and policies will determine if we can deliver quality care or not. While we don't describe the technicalities of the build—much of it is done by the vendor and invisible to clinical staff—we describe the impact of those technicalities on the realities of patient care and on the way the system is used (or not used) by physicians and nurses.

BIG-BANG VERSUS SEQUENTIAL CONVERSION

In the run-up to conversion, the earliest issue to arise pertains to overall strategy: Do we do a big-bang or a sequential conversion? This issue actually entails two questions because the choice of big-bang versus sequential conversion can pertain to either the EHR functions (e.g., CPOE, documentation) or the "geographic" areas of the hospital in which we bring up these functions (e.g., the ED, L&D, the clinics). We have two choices:

1. We can implement viewing, CPOE, and documentation all at once (i.e., big-bang conversion) or in phases (e.g., first

viewing, then CPOE, and finally documentation, each a separate phase and a separate conversion event).

2. We can convert the entire facility at one time or divide it by location in the hospital (e.g., first the ED, then the inpatient wards, and finally the clinics, each a separate phase and a separate conversion event).

Functional Phases

Most hospitals—often for historical rather than purely logical reasons—have started with an initial conversion phase enabling the viewing of data, implemented CPOE second, and then finished with a documentation phase. There have been innumerable variants of this theme, particularly with regard to nurse order entry versus physician order entry. In many cases, once the catalog is ready for use, pharmacists enter medication orders in the first phase, ward secretaries enter most orders and nurses enter medications in the second phase, and then the sequence finishes with physician order entry. Sequencing has become more rapid and truncated in recent years as EHRs become more common and physicians become accustomed to using CPOE, and many hospitals are converting directly from paper orders to full CPOE all at once. There is little risk to launching CPOE simultaneously for pharmacists, nurses, and physicians other than the standard caveats discussed in previous chapters, such as design and policy considerations and the need to have a fully functional catalog, appropriate OEFs, and optimal order set design.

There is still considerable disagreement as to whether it is preferable to have physicians begin CPOE and electronic documentation simultaneously or in two separate phases. Several considerations play a role in this decision, including the cost of having two conversions, the stress involved for physicians, the previous experience of the staff, vendors' recommendations (which vary between and even within vendors), and the workflow flexibility of the function itself (see discussion on partial conversion of documentation later in this chapter).

Cost considerations may be paramount, but they can work in either direction. On the one hand, two separate conversions can be more expensive if they require that the same support staff be used twice. On the other hand, in some institutions, separating the conversions can actually **decrease** cost by allowing the hospital to amortize the cost of the support staff over a greater time span and thus use their resources more effectively. For a hypothetical example, if each conversion requires 30 support staff, and the hospital has only these 30 staff available but a single, large conversion would require more than the current 30 staff, it may be cheaper to separate the two events (using the 30 support staff twice) rather than find additional FTEs to support the single conversion. Solutions are seldom so simple, however. Typically, a hospital must look at outside consultant costs, per diem staff, sister hospitals from which experienced staff can be borrowed for subsequent conversions, vendor support costs, contract timelines, regulatory deadlines, and other factors.

Geographic Phases

Implementation in geographic phases—separate conversions for different areas of the hospital—is also fairly common and (with a great deal of care and forethought) can be successful and allow the hospital to test the adequacy of the build and make improvements before taking the system hospital-wide. However, risk arises when patients move between two locations, of which one has CPOE and one does not. In the worst-case scenario, a ward in which some patients have paper records and others have electronic records is a recipe for patient injury and malpractice. In such cases, nurses are often uncertain as to which patients have paper medication lists and paper orders and which have electronic medication administration records (MARs) and electronic orders. The result is duplicated orders, missed orders, and confusion about medications, therapies, and labs.

Geographic phases always pose risks when patients move from a CPOE venue to a paper venue or vice versa. The surest way of minimizing this risk is to find venues where transfer is either unlikely (e.g., L&D patients are unlikely to be transferred to a medical ward) or similar to a discharge and where staff are already careful

---

Never Split a Single Ward into Two Groups of Patients

In one odd case, two large, urban hospitals—one dedicated to cancer care and one largely to gynecologic care—were located on the same block, and their buildings were attached. They were separate corporations and had separate wards, staffs, policies, and medical records. On one ward, however, for largely historical reasons, they still had mingled beds, half the patients belonging to hospital A and half to hospital B. As difficult as this situation was, hospital A elected to convert to an EHR while hospital B firmly intended to remain on paper. The initial decision was to include half the patients on the shared ward in the EHR and leave the other half on paper.

The vendor and the hospitals' attorneys, quality assurance departments, and nursing staffs forced a reconsideration of this policy, concerned that nurses would have a difficult time telling which patients were which and that the policy would put patients at high risk (as well as cause frustration among the nursing staffs).

The final policy was that—regardless of the hospital to which the patient was officially admitted—all patients on the combined ward would be included in the EHR. The conversion progressed well, although issues remained when patients were transferred from the EHR ward to a paper-based ward.

when moving patients between geographic venues (e.g., ED patients being transferred to an inpatient bed status). As long as workflow is carefully planned, other types of geographic phasing, such as converting only the ICU and then later converting the remainder of the hospital, can also be considered—and have been accomplished successfully. In every case in which geographic phasing is used, the major risks are the same: lost orders, duplicate orders, and confusion about patients' medications (and allergies, procedures, and so on), particularly their MARs.

If a single location is the first conversion site, it usually is the ED. Separating out the ED is common; other venues, including L&D, the ICU, outpatient clinics, and specialty wards, have also been converted first, but this strategy is less common. In many cases, the OR is not initially included due to the issues involved in the transfer of care (from the ward to the OR, from the OR to the PACU, and then back to the ward) but considered (and converted) separately, and only after the remainder of the hospital has finished converting. A final exception is oncology wards, due to the difficulty inherent in managing the complexity and timing of oncology orders and the constraints imposed by dosing, interactions, lifetime exposure, and the narrow therapeutic windows of many interventions.

Partial Conversions

In certain situations, use of CPOE may not be optimal due to either the workflow or the nature of the functions available, and exceptions to the use of CPOE are made. Often these exceptions constitute long-term policy, so conversions are not so much partial as they are complete with allowances made for special medical circumstances in which patient care might be better served by verbal orders. Although at least one hospital has attempted a policy of full CPOE with no exceptions of any kind, most hospitals have felt that certain exceptions are consistent with good medical care. The following situations are the three most common exceptions:

1. **Codes:** Many hospitals have exempted both medical and trauma codes, allowing verbal and written orders to be used in such events. In some hospitals, orders (particularly medication orders) must later be transcribed into the computer to ensure that the MAR is accurate for later medical decision making; in other hospitals, these events remain on paper. Perhaps unexpectedly, there has been a growing movement to stop exempting codes from the requirement of CPOE. This shift tends to occur a year or so after hospitals (and medical staff) become used to CPOE, finding it simpler to enter the orders immediately than to reconcile paper to computer afterwards. This trend is more common among hospitals in which clinical staff use portable computers on wheels or handheld tablets to enter orders.
2. **Surgery or cases in which physicians are not available:** This exception includes both surgeons in the operating room and physicians performing procedures. In almost all cases, the exception is based on the principle of best patient care and requires that an exception be made in any situation in which physicians are gloved or otherwise involved in emergent care and an immediate order is needed to deliver good patient care.
3. **No access to a computer:** This exception includes cases in which physicians are neither in the hospital nor in their offices but in their cars, at home, or at nonmedical locations. The principle is that it is easier for nurses to place orders than for physicians to do so, and patient care will be faster and safer overall as a result, assuming that the nurses read back verbal orders to the ordering physician for confirmation as required by The Joint Commission.

Partial conversions can also occur strategically in the case of documentation. This case is markedly different from CPOE, which cannot be done on a partial basis without posing substantial risk to patient safety. For example, it would be risky in the extreme if

- a physician had both CPOE patients and patients with paper orders, or
- a patient had some CPOE orders and some paper orders.

Partial conversion of documentation—while not usually recommended—has often been done successfully. In many cases, hospitals have encouraged electronic documentation at conversion but required it only after several days or weeks have passed. This sort of partial conversion has taken several forms:

- Physicians are required to document a certain minimum number of patients electronically each day, and this requirement gradually increases.
- Physicians are encouraged to document electronically but permitted to use other methods if stressed, and this loophole is gradually closed.
- Certain physicians pilot electronic documentation, and it is gradually extended to the entire medical staff.

While partial CPOE puts patients' safety at high risk, the risk of partial electronic documentation is lower, becoming an issue only when physicians (or other clinicians) are having a hard time finding prior documents on their patients. They may, for example, have to search two locations in a record for a previous dictation or a previous electronic template document, thereby slowing the delivery of medical care. This risk may be outweighed by increased ease of adoption, in that physicians find conversion less stressful and have more time to transition to the new workflow.

Recommendation: Whenever feasible, a big-bang approach is recommended. It is increasingly becoming the norm, although exceptions still abound.

SCHEDULING THE CONVERSION

Finding a day and time for the conversion is far less important than keeping it. While most hospitals put considerable effort into choosing a conversion date that will cause the least disruption, and while there are many legitimate reasons to alter the planned conversion date, there are significant costs to changing this date. **Rule one: Never change the conversion date.**

The most obvious cost incurred by changing dates is financial, but the most important cost is political. The financial cost might be unexpected, but it should be predictable and avoidable. When conversion dates change, not only are there contractual costs; it also is often difficult (and even impossible in rare cases) to ensure sufficient support staff for the new date. Vendors usually have calendars predicated on long lead times (i.e., several months) for their consulting or support staff. Changes to their calendars either cannot be made or, if they can be made, occasion a substantial increase in costs. The closer to go-live a postponement occurs, the higher the costs. **Rule two: If you change the conversion date, change it early in the project.**

The political costs of changing the date of a conversion are enormous and cannot be overly stressed. Not only does the project staff become upset; in many cases hospitals also find that their vendors—once helpful and supportive—have suddenly become grudging and unresponsive. And who can blame them? No one—vendor or hospital—wants a partner who reneges on a commitment, however crucial the need to do so, and one can scarcely be expected to trust the other's word a second time. The largest political costs, however, accrue from the loss of credibility among the clinical staff. Physicians who have been given "firm dates" several times in a row roll their eyes when that firm date changes yet again, or worse yet, they simply ignore the new date altogether. **Rule three: If you change the conversion date, never change it twice.**

Case Study

Eight weeks prior to go-live, the CNO of a large, urban hospital (with an ED volume of 90,000 annual visits) called a meeting and overrode all previous decisions made by the ED nursing staff regarding ED nursing documentation. The CNO hadn't attended any of the previous design meetings, nor had she been willing to review the staff's decisions; she simply had given generic approval. During the meeting, she declined the ED nursing staff's offers to explain the rationale of their decisions. To meet the CNO's demand would have cost an extra $60,000 (which was not included in the project contract) and pushed the conversion date back five weeks because it would have required that all training and programming be put on hold while the changes were made and then redone once the revisions were in place. In addition, it would have undercut the credibility of the project. The CEO reversed the CNO's decision, the conversion went ahead as originally scheduled, and while the credibility of the project was not undermined, that of the CNO certainly was, and she was later fired.

When scheduling a conversion, project teams should reasonably consider patient load. In most cases, conversion occurs over a weekend, but Monday mornings are not uncommonly chosen. The most common window for a conversion is anywhere from midnight to 8 a.m. However, the optimum time for a conversion should not be based on the national or historical norm but on the needs of the hospital.

For an ED conversion, the time should be based on the predicted nadir in patient volume and available supplemental staff (as well as staff who would normally be scheduled at the time of conversion), ancillary support (radiology, lab, pharmacy), and

Want a Reputation for Unreliability (and perhaps dishonesty)?

For various reasons, including financial necessities, difficulties with the build, unexpected staff shortages, and a new CEO, a large, western hospital had changed its conversion date from January to March, then to April, and finally to August. In each case, there was a rationale supporting the necessity and unavoidability of the change, and each time it was carefully explained to the clinical staffs throughout the hospital.

By July, the project team was no longer able to convince the staff physicians to attend training. In several cases, the physicians actually laughed and hung up on the trainers. They listened to the (new) CEO's pleas more politely during the next general staff meeting but still ignored his appeal. On the day of conversion, less than 10 percent of the medical staff had even seen a trainer in seven months let alone completed the training. Only a handful of physicians had up-to-date, active passwords. More than 90 percent of the nursing staff had been trained, but few had taken the training seriously. Polls showed that less than 5 percent of the nurses and none of the physicians had believed that the conversion would take place in August.

The actual conversion lasted less than two hours. The physicians didn't even bother complaining about the system; they simply ignored both the system and the support staff. They continued to use paper orders, and the system had to be shut down.

The ultimate cost of the project was well over twice the initial projection, and a year later, the system was still inactive.

any other local issues. While a weekend may be the best choice for a med-surg floor, it may be the worst choice for most EDs. Likewise, the time of year can have an enormous impact on the success of a conversion. In many hospitals in Florida, the census may more than double over the winter (as compared to the summer) season, prompting the decision to choose a low-census month for a conversion, such as July. The arrival of new staff—such as residents in early July—may also have an impact on the date.

Patient Scheduling

While the project team should consider the patient census, available clinical and support staff, and other details when setting the optimal date for conversion, any date can be accommodated by adjusting staffing and patient scheduling. The most common considerations are the surgery schedule and the clinic schedule. While there is no rule of thumb—both depend on how stressed the staff are currently, how many elective procedures are done, and the internal politics of each department—many hospitals have cut back patient load significantly during conversion. In some cases, all elective surgeries are postponed for one to two weeks, and the normal load in the OR and clinics is commonly cut back by 20 to 25 percent. A number of hospitals have felt that they were sufficiently comfortable with the system (and with their staffs) to maintain the OR and clinic schedules without any change whatsoever, although they increased the support staff (largely super-users) during the initial week of conversion.

As a general rule, the OR and clinics are the only two areas that can alter their patient load. Departments that cannot do so, such as L&D and the ED, focus on support rather than patient volume.

PRELOADING DATA

Almost all hospitals have a carefully designed plan to preload clinical data. In general, these data are of two types: (1) those essential for current patient care and (2) historical data that are desirable to have but not critical. The former—current patients' medications, allergies, orders, laboratory data, radiology results, and MARs— are generally preloaded one to two days (and often within the 12 hours) prior to conversion. These data, which encompass the records of current patients since admission, are required to treat patients and have a direct impact on medical decision making on the day of conversion. This information must be available at go-live. It can be difficult to add orders and medications made in the last few hours or minutes prior to bringing up the new system. In an early-morning conversion, this task usually occupies a number of staff during the last few hours of the night.

The latter data—patient histories, discharge summaries, progress notes, and medical documentation in general (especially documentation from previous admissions)—have a lower clinical priority. Most hospitals—depending on human and financial resources—load prior documents into the system, but only those created after a specified date, such as documents dated within the past six months or the past two years. While clinical documentation from several years ago may be desirable to have—and even necessary in some cases—it is less likely to have an impact on current care, and loading it will cost extra. Many hospitals leave data (e.g., prior radiology readings) on an incompatible EHR they implemented in the past, maintaining dual portals for clinical access, sometimes even indefinitely. This process—adding historical documentation—should be started prior to conversion. In many cases, hospitals continue to enter large bodies of information into the EHR over the first few months or more after conversion.

SUPPORTING THE CONVERSION

All conversions need support. In general, support consists of superusers who are present on the wards, but it should also consist of telephone support, emotional support, and the unseen support provided by the analysts and programmers who make changes as required. Most hospitals provide separate support for the physician staff, usually by giving them access to a special physician phone line and having physicians without clinical responsibilities present in the hospital.

In the past, the issue of physician support often included the question of financial or other incentives. Although such incentives are becoming uncommon, the issue still surfaces among hospital-owned practices because the physicians are required to use the hospital's new system, and adoption may have a direct—if temporary—negative impact on their income. Some hospitals have given financial guarantees to these physicians, often for a limited period, such as the first month or two after conversion. But many hospitals are leery of providing such guarantees, arguing that they encourage physicians to take it easy and not make a good effort to learn to use the new system. A few hospitals have structured their guarantees by offering a minimum figure to all the physicians (to prevent complaints about the initial period of learning) and then additional rewards for those who become efficient users quickly. Although such guarantees are becoming less common as EHRs become more common, they are worth considering.

Ratio and Levels of Support

The number of support staff, not surprisingly, varies with circumstances, but the mean support ratio is 15 users per one support staff member. *Support staff* refers to the number of super-users who are present on the clinical floors and does not include those who are restricted to the command center, analysts, programmers, or managers (unless they are offering direct support). More support staff are needed in high-intensity areas, such as the ED, PACU, and ICU. Fewer are needed at night or during times of low patient volume, such as weekends in the OR.

Clinicians (as opposed to ward secretaries, for example) should be given preferred access to clinical support staff. The same is recommended for other clinical staff: Nurses should have preferred access to nursing support staff, pharmacists to pharmacist support staff, and so on. Such pairings are not always feasible, in which case preference should be given to support staff who have some clinical background, good social skills, and the best understanding of a particular workflow. There are examples of nonclinical personnel who have been remarkably adept at offering support to physicians and nurses, generally due to superb social skills.

Those offering direct support must have backup. Backup can take one of three forms of increasing importance. For example, if a nonclinical or nonphysician super-user is attempting to support a physician—particularly an irate one—with little success, the super-user should be able to call on backup, in this order:

1. A physician-specific help line that can provide immediate, real-time support
2. A clinically adept physician who can offer further support, generally because he or she is familiar with the system and has used it to deliver patient care
3. A high-level physician administrator (e.g., CMO) who can adequately address political or personality issues raised by physicians

These same levels of support pertain to nursing staff (i.e., a nurse-specific help line, another clinical nurse, and the nurse manager or CNO) and other clinical users.

Change Control

Change control—a systematic approach to managing EHR modification—must always respond to two opposing needs: (1) the need for a rapid response to clinical problems with the build and (2) a responsible, carefully vetted solution that does not introduce complications or errors into the system or workflow. All change control must be documented and overseen by someone at the C-suite or program manager level. This individual must have a firm appreciation of both clinical priorities and system capabilities; both are crucial to making an appropriate decision. This dual role is often filled by CMIOs because they have both clinical and technical responsibilities. The leader is assisted by an aide, who maintains a record of all requests, their priorities, their resource needs, and their current status. The aide's role is as important as that of the decision maker.

Priority equals clinical importance divided by the resources required. At first sight, most command centers would establish priorities solely on the basis of two risks: immediate risk to patient safety and immediate financial risk. While this perspective is understandable and a good place to start, these priorities must be balanced against the required (and available) resources. Some issues may be of low importance, but because so few resources are required to resolve them, they should be considered high priority and addressed immediately. Other issues may be of far higher importance than these "trivial fixes," but the resources needed to resolve them may be so substantial that they may not be addressed for several days.

An actual example of an issue that lent itself to a trivial fix in one hospital was a staff complaint that the word *pneumonia* was misspelled in the name of an order set. This issue was of low importance, but only a moment was required to correct it, and the solution introduced no risk to the system. This issue was made a high priority and fixed within an hour of go-live.

An example of an issue of high importance would be a staff complaint that the entire insulin protocol is erroneous and needs to be rewritten from scratch; it contains gross clinical errors and risks patient safety as it stands. Several hours of physician, nursing, and pharmacist time would be required to redesign the insulin protocol, and then the order set would need to be corrected in the build. This time-consuming, resource-intensive solution may be given lower priority, done a day or two after go-live while—as a temporary workaround—the nursing staff rely on the old paper form of the insulin protocol.

While these two exceptions—the trivial fix and the resource-intensive clinical need—often occur, the general, more common rule of thumb is that clinical (and to a lesser extent financial) issues take priority. Put simply, the list of issues is generally ruled by clinical priority.

As in most complex social settings, perception is often as important as reality. In the typical conversion, especially when there is resistance by clinical users, communication is key to success. If you solve a problem, tell the person who complained and the rest of the staff as well. If you can't solve a problem, say so and explain why. If it will take two days to solve a problem, let people know the time frame. While you can't promise results, you can inform the user. In most cases, users have no idea about (and little interest in) what the support staff are doing in the command center. What they care about passionately is their ability to provide patient care and to get their work done. You don't need to explain **how** the system works, but you do need to explain **when** the system will work. No solution is complete unless you have given feedback to the user who raised the issue.

Always tell clinical staff what you are doing about their issues. No matter what miracles you accomplish, clinical staff always assume that you aren't fixing the issue unless you tell them so. Tell them what you are doing, tell them when you expect to solve the issue, and tell them again when you have fixed the issue. Don't just solve problems; communicate everything you do.

Change control follows a typical and predictable time course. The rate of change to the build is slow and steady, decreasing almost to zero just prior to the conversion as the build is locked down to ensure a stable, reliable system. Immediately after conversion (the first week), the rate of change increases because a number of errors and potential improvements become obvious. Change control is rapid, and all requests are considered in real-time or within a matter of hours, and decisions and action immediately follow if change is appropriate. As the rate of change falls again to a stable level in the weeks after conversion, change control takes on a thoughtful, committee format in which written suggestions from users may be required, followed by study, consensus, committee voting, referral to other hospital groups, and final decision and action.

Although a rapid change control process is typical and appropriate in the first few days after conversion, it does not abrogate the need for documentation and due consideration; it merely requires that issues be documented and considered immediately and efficiently. It is characterized by quick decisions and immediate actions, not by undocumented requests and knee-jerk reactions.

During most conversions, the command center personnel meet twice daily, although this schedule tapers off after the first week or so, and meetings become a daily event. Decisions are not postponed until the next meeting, however. The command center leader—for example, the CMIO—must be available to make decisions in real-time throughout the day and must have a representative who makes decisions at night. The meetings serve as a forum for communicating the decisions that have been made since the previous meeting and the overall state of the conversion. These updates are usually communicated by role (i.e., physicians, nurses, pharmacists) as well as by unit (e.g., ED, L&D, med-surg). While these meetings are intended to convey information both "upward" (to the leaders) and "downward" (to the support staff and super-users), they also bind the team members together emotionally and help them catch problems that they might otherwise overlook. Most hospitals also construct an

---

Example of an Executive Summary Outline
from a Major Urban Hospital Chain

- Conversion status: project leader
  - The front door (access, registration, what are patients saying?)
  - Turnaround times (ED, transfers, OR, pharmacy)
  - Impact on core process
- Physicians: CMO
  - The "pulse" of the physicians (i.e., how the physicians feel about the conversion)
  - Super-user engagement
  - Resident utilization
  - Physician utilization detail
- Patient care delivery: CNO
  - Shift report updates
  - Clinical technical team decisions
  - The learning curve
  - Ancillary impacts
- System issues: CIO
  - Issues management
  - Critical changes to the system

---

executive summary that not only conveys the information needed by the CEO and other C-suite-level administrators but also succinctly communicates the status of the conversion. Such summaries should include figures (e.g., percentage of CPOE usage) whenever available as well as the number of open issues, the proposed solutions to those issues, the number of closed issues, and any issues that could put patients at significant risk.

Duration of Support

Support usually is highest for a week or two after conversion, but the baseline level of support needed after this initial period is still higher than that needed prior to conversion. In special cases, support may be minimal, perhaps only a few days in the case of conversions that merely add a few features to an already familiar system. In other cases, support may remain at a high level for a month or more, as in cases when the conversion encompasses major changes and staff are markedly resistant. Support is often tailored not only to the clinical role (i.e., physician or nurse) but also to the system. For example, when introducing both CPOE and a voice recognition system for documentation, specific support for voice recognition is often provided by outside consultants in addition to CPOE support.

Typically, hospitals ensure 24-hours-a-day, at-the-elbow support for the first week; day shift support for the following week (and phone support for the night shift); and phone support thereafter. Support must be available on an as-needed but permanent basis for newly hired physicians, *locum tenens* providers, visiting consultants, and similar clinical personnel who will require training and support in the future.

Stress levels post-conversion are predictable and rise to three successive peaks. The first peak occurs on the first day after conversion and is typified by emotional outbursts, but it is tempered by a common feeling of "being in this together" and supporting a common team effort. The second peak always occurs on the third or fourth day after conversion and is typified by fatigue and the sudden realization that the user is really going to have to live with the system, warts and all. Users may have been feeling heroic and priding themselves on supporting the team, but they are now tired and disgruntled. The third peak occurs several weeks after conversion, when users' issues are no longer handled within hours or days but must be submitted to a committee of their peers for consensual review and deliberation—and acted on only after several weeks or months. Many users get used to rapid resolution of their issues and begin to feel that no one is listening or that the vendor (or the hospital's own IT department) has left them "high and dry."

Problems and Solutions

Conversions have typical problems. On the first day, the three Ps—privileges, passwords, and printers—are almost always major reasons staff call the command center help line. Within minutes of go-live, it is predictable that users will call to find out why they can't see the right interface or are unable to perform their necessary functions. The two most typical issues with privileges are

1. the user still has old privileges and has not been granted new privileges, and
2. the user has not been granted the correct new privileges.

The latter is typical of midlevel providers, such as nurse practitioners who should have been granted CPOE privileges but have been granted only routine nursing privileges.

The issue of passwords is usually user error; the user has simply forgotten his new password or has not reset his password for the new system. Occasionally, the error is present in the system files or occurs when the trainer did not reset the user's password at the time he certified the user as having been trained. In both cases, the response to the problem should be immediate; the issue is not difficult for an efficient command center staff to resolve.

The issue of printers is universal. Often a printer simply has not been assigned to the user's device, or the wrong printer has been assigned. Contributing to this problem are confusing, nonintuitive interfaces that must be navigated to assign a printer. Moreover, most hospitals use arcane naming conventions for their printers, making it difficult to identify the correct printer other than by copying the printer name carefully and by rote. The issues of privileges and passwords are transient, seldom arising beyond the first day of conversion, but printer issues often last a week or more, over which users' frustration and complaints gradually decrease.

Two other issues cause predictable frustration for users, often well after the initial few days of conversion: medication reconciliation and the discharge process. In the most successful hospital conversions, an inordinate amount of resources—investments in workflow analysis, formulary matching, training, communication, and support—have been allocated to these two recurrent obstacles. It helps to point out that the requirement for medication reconciliation is not imposed by the EHR itself (i.e., the vendor) but by meaningful use (i.e., governmental regulation) and that medication reconciliation has always been a routine part of good medical care. Physicians have always tried to ensure that the nursing staff and the patient are aware of exactly which medications the patient is taking and which have been discontinued. This process has also been a standard part of physician-to-physician transfer. With conversion and meaningful use, however, the requirement to do meds rec in an EHR has changed the workflow and has often increased the difficulty of that workflow, generally due to poorly designed interfaces and the problem of formulary mismatching. The result is a better reconciliation for the patient, but at the cost of increasing physicians' time loss and frustration.

The discharge process is likewise a victim of interfaces that inadequately reflect the clinical workflow, contain unnecessary information, require unnecessary clicking, and slow patient care. While this process can and almost certainly will be improved as vendors and physicians strive to improve clinical workflow as well as patient

If You Don't Give Users Privileges to Order,
You Risk Patient Care

A large, academic hospital on the west coast of Florida had just gone live and was having problems in L&D. A young mother, delivering her first child, needed Pitocin immediately, but the nurse practitioner was unable to order the medication from the pharmacy. The clinical staff were angry, the patient was waiting, and the command center had already put the nurse practitioner on hold once. When the right person finally got on the line, it took only moments to grant her the correct provider privileges (she had been listed as having nurse, rather than nurse practitioner, privileges). Listing the incorrect midlevel privileges had wasted time, caused frustration, and put the patient at totally avoidable risk.

Lesson: Review all privileges, especially of midlevel staff, and ensure a rapid response to problems with privileges on the day of conversion.

safety, there is seldom any effective way of easing this burden at the time of conversion. As is the case with medication reconciliation, the most successful hospitals have accepted the current limits of their systems and have focused on workflows, training, communication, and user support.

MEASURING SUCCESS

There are numerous examples of using the wrong measures of patient care as quality indicators during EHR conversions. One such inadequate measure is length of stay (LOS) in the ED. Some hospitals naïvely assume that decreased LOS is an indicator of quality and a worthwhile goal in itself during conversion: Shorter LOS equals improved patient care. One hospital that we worked with strove with might and main to reduce its mean LOS from six hours to four hours. As discussed earlier in this book, there is danger behind this simple goal: If shorter LOS is our only (or our primary) goal, we can easily reduce LOS to a matter of minutes by restricting our actions to simply registering the patient, collecting billing information, and then discharging the patient without further ado.

This absurd example underscores why we should be shocked and concerned when a hospital states that its goal is solely to reduce LOS—which many hospitals do. With appropriate caveats, LOS might serve as a very useful **marker**, but as the only marker, reduced LOS is a misleading, risky goal. We should be asking about the overall quality of care delivered, not solely the time it took to deliver that care, independent of its quality. The overall quality might well **include** a short LOS, but we can scarcely defend LOS as a single indicator of the quality of the patient care we deliver.

The same is true of all measures of success. Such measures should be seen as potentially flawed but honest attempts to assess the underlying quality of patient care. They should be

1. realistic, sophisticated indicators of the quality of care;
2. objective and measurable; and
3. amenable to change and improvement.

The first characteristic has already been addressed earlier in the book: Every measure should be taken with a grain of salt and must be seen in a larger clinical context rather than as an independent measure of quality. The second characteristic requires that useful measures not be subjective or ill defined. For example, data indicating that ten patients described their care as "good" are of little use as a measure of the quality of care. On the other hand, data indicating that the average "door-to-doctor" time is 55 minutes are useful and objective. The third characteristic requires that we be capable of changing the measure. Simply showing that 30 percent of patients present with pediatric problems is not a measure of success because we have no control over it. Regulations, financial limitations, and reality put boundaries on what we can attain, and it is fruitless to measure the inevitable.

A final characteristic of measures of success is desirable but not always feasible. The best measures of success are gathered prior to and after conversion, thereby showing improvement. In some cases, the absence of an electronic system may preclude an accurate measure of what we were doing prior to conversion, and we may have to fall back on two sets of incompatible data ("apples and

---

Actual Data from a Large Southern Academic Center

- Clinic support numbers:
  - —One person for the front desk
  - —One person for the nonphysician clinical staff
  - —One person for each provider (or clinical team)
  - —One support team leader for each clinic
- Duration of support:
  - —Full support for weeks 1–2, 50 percent support for weeks 3–4, and then a single person per clinic for weeks 5–6
- Patient scheduling:
  - —We scheduled only 50 percent of the normal load for weeks 1–2, then 75 percent for weeks 3–4. Those who did not reduce their schedules had problems meeting the patient load. A few clinics that reduced their schedules were able to increase them more quickly than planned.
- Preloading data:
  - —The hospital paid for moonlighting residents and nurses to preload meds, allergies, problem lists, and procedure histories.

---

oranges") or rely on post-conversion trending to suggest continual improvement. For example, if we want to measure the success of allergy alerts in preventing patient medication errors, we cannot reliably compare prior rates of error to post-conversion rates of error because the measurements themselves have changed, as well as the data. If we can at least show that the use of such alerts is gradually but steadily decreasing error rates (regardless of the uncertain error rate prior to conversion), we can still make the case that we have successfully lowered medication errors.

KEY POINTS

- Should conversions be done all at once or in pieces?
  —When feasible, a big-bang conversion is preferable to conversion in sequential stages.
  —If dividing implementation by units, consider converting the ED, clinics, or L&D first.
  —Avoid partial conversions.
- When scheduling the conversion
  —never change the conversion date;
  —choose a week, day, and time that will cause the least stress for users; and
  —decrease the patient load if feasible (i.e., clinics, elective surgeries).
- Recommendations for conversion support include the following:
  —Fifteen users per super-user is a good default ratio.
  —Set up a physician help line, and provide at-the-elbow physician support.
  —Provide 24/7 support for at least one to two weeks.
- Guidelines for change control include the following:
  —Track all issues, and make decisions rapidly.
  —Priority equals clinical importance divided by resources required.
  —Tell users what you are going to do, are doing, and have done.

CHAPTER 11

Optimization

If you optimize everything, you will always be unhappy.

—*Donald Knuth*

AFTER CONVERSION, EMPHASIS shifts from implementation to optimization. *Optimization* has various meanings, but it generally refers to

- the initial tweaking that occurs immediately post-implementation, and
- the ongoing, permanent process that is part of EHR improvement.

INITIAL OPTIMIZATION

The initial tweaking that occurs post-implementation has been a universal response in all successful hospitals. It includes change control, error correction, and workflow redesign. Generally, this phase of optimization is a response to previously unrecognized errors in design and implementation but also includes retraining clinical personnel to improve their ability to use the system and fine-tuning clinical use. Retraining typically includes a review of macros, filters, and favorites folders. Even in the best of cases, users tend to slide over or forget parts of their initial training; retraining catches these omissions and enables users to become more efficient. To use a common analogy, initial training teaches users to ride a bicycle, and retraining teaches them to pop wheelies, shift gears, and race at full speed.

Beyond training issues, hospitals usually discover unexpected problems with policies, procedures, and workflows that were not predicted (and perhaps not predictable) prior to implementation but became obvious and important once conversion occurred.

ONGOING OPTIMIZATION

Optimization refers to far more than the necessity to tweak the system immediately post-conversion. Hospitals that have successfully completed an initial implementation (e.g., CPOE) find there

---

If You Can't Find It, You Can't Order It

A large, national chain had instituted a series of conversions in its several-dozen hospitals over a seven-year period, using a uniform build, catalog, and order sets. It hired consultants to determine why it was still having adoption problems even after prolonged use. After several years of CPOE, 3 × 5 index cards listing the nonintuitive names of common orderables were still taped to the monitors of almost every computer to assist users. Order sets had remained unchanged since conversion, and many of them contained medications no longer on the formulary. The EHR had been kept up to date with the latest available version from the vendor, as had the hardware, but almost no effort had been put into optimizing the orderables, the order sets, or any other user-related issue. As one user put it succinctly, "I could probably order it faster than ever, if I could just find the order in the first place."

---

is an opportunity (and a need) for continual improvement, not only in the system but in how they **use** the system.

This type of optimization—continual optimization—is now occupying center stage worldwide as hospitals attempt to refine and improve their use of the EHRs they have already installed. Typically, hospitals already are using CPOE and electronic documentation and now are entering the phase of ongoing, permanent efforts to optimize their EHRs. Continual optimization has five aspects:

1. Installing EHR solutions that are available but not yet in use
2. Keeping up to date with technical improvements
3. Keeping up to date with regulatory and financial requirements and recommendations
4. Keeping up to date with the latest evidence-based clinical standards
5. Optimizing clinical use of the EHR

The last aspect—optimizing clinical use—is the key issue at successful hospitals and is discussed in detail later in this chapter. It demands clinical perspective and has a direct impact on the quality of patient care.

Installing EHR Solutions That Are Available but Not Yet in Use

The first of these five aspects encompasses the installation of solutions offered by the EHR vendor that the hospital has not yet used. Hospitals may implement only portions of the available suite of functions initially, such as CPOE, and then add electronic documentation later, or they may use the EHR for their wards and then later add surgical functions. This sort of add-on, whether for ambulatory clinics, pediatrics, oncology, women's health, surgery, documentation, or other functions, occurs in hospitals that already have some practical experience with their EHRs. Most add-ons are installed early in the implementation process, and hospitals may choose to install additional solutions later as vendors add new functions to their existing systems. For example, we foresee the addition of word recognition software for verbal orders in the near future. Additional thought and planning will be required to install this solution, but it will—in a sense—optimize current functionality.

Keeping Up to Date with Technical Improvements

The second aspect of continual optimization depends on whether the vendor makes and offers technical improvements. These types of improvements are incremental and enhance functions that have already been installed. In most cases, these enhancements require little adaptation on the part of users. For example, most vendors are continually improving their interfaces, making it easier for the user to extract information, find and place orders, and document meaningful medical information. Current interfaces are still inadequate for efficient clinical use, not because they are not designed intelligently and carefully but because **they still are not optimized for real-world clinical use**. Designers still make inaccurate assumptions regarding which data to emphasize, how orders are placed, and the actual purposes of documentation. For example, most vendors still assume that the purpose of physician documentation is only to document data when in fact the purpose is to document the patient's story and explain the implications of the data and the rationale for clinical decisions. These and other similar assumptions are gradually being replaced by more careful attention to appropriate information regarding clinical workflow and the actual needs of patient care. While technical improvements have a direct impact on clinical use, hospitals—by and large—passively depend on their vendors to make such enhancements and generally are unable to drive such enhancements directly.

Keeping Up to Date with Regulatory and Financial Requirements and Recommendations

The third aspect—keeping up to date with current regulatory and financial requirements and recommendations for medical care—depends on the actions of regulatory bodies, insurers, government payers, and international organizations as well as on the ability of the EHR vendor to quickly and effectively respond to them. While this type of optimization often has an impact on both the quality of patient care and the clinical workflow, it is generally reactive rather than proactive. For example, with regard to the venous thromboembolism (VTE) prophylaxis guideline issued by the Institute for Clinical Systems Improvement (ICSI) (National Guideline Clearinghouse 2012), vendors might develop a tool that helps hospitals follow the recommendations. A hospital can optimize its response to externally imposed requirements and recommendations in only two ways: by using the tools developed by its EHR vendor for this purpose and by changing the workflow of its clinical staff.

> ### *If You Build It*—and Make It Easy to Use—*They Will Come*
>
> A large community hospital on the gulf coast of Florida was the first client to install its EHR vendor's initial software package designed to help the hospital comply with the ICSI's recommendations for VTE prophylaxis. The installation was done flawlessly, but user compliance was almost zero for the first two months. The hospital worked with the vendor to optimize the VTE interface, paying particular attention to when the VTE screen popped up in the physician workflow and to how the interface could most easily permit documentation of VTE exceptions. User compliance climbed immediately and remained almost universal.

Keeping Up to Date with the Latest Evidence-Based Clinical Standards

The fourth aspect—keeping up to date with best practices, particularly with current standards of evidence-based medicine—is again for most hospitals largely a response to externally imposed standards. Even large, academic hospitals can drive only a limited, narrow set of such standards as leaders and accepted sources of best practices. Most standards are national or global rather than local and generally cannot be determined independently by any one hospital. The need to remain current with external standards has prompted EHR vendors to develop services that offer the latest information on best practices and help incorporate these standards into EHRs. Some EHR vendors (e.g., Zynx, ProVation, and BMJ) offer commercial order sets that reflect current standards and link orderables to current references and supportive medical literature. This facet of optimization is certainly a key part of quality patient care, but it demands little from hospitals other than appropriate vendor contracts and regular attention from those overseeing optimization.

Optimizing Clinical Use of the EHR

The fifth aspect—optimizing the clinical use of the EHR—demands a great deal of expertise and creativity. In practice, this type of optimization is most critical for the majority of hospitals.

Optimization is not merely a matter of finding better ways of meeting your current goals but also includes finding new and better goals. Done well, optimization is not a goal to achieve but an ongoing process of achieving excellence. Goals change, and optimization continues withal.

The overall vision—improving patient care—remains, but the paths we take and the methods we use to improve patient care change continually, as they must. The EHR is a new tool to help us achieve an old goal. Most hospitals have specific goals that stand in for this overall vision, such as attaining Magnet status, becoming a Level 1 trauma center, or achieving better Press Ganey scores. Each of these goals must be reevaluated and must change with time. The hospital that picks a small number of narrow goals, accomplishes these goals, and then rests on its laurels soon becomes unsuccessful. While specific goals are important, all are merely markers toward better patient care; none of the goals themselves is better patient care. The successful hospital defines specific goals, meets those goals, and then defines new goals in an ongoing effort to deliver better care.

No hospital can attain its goals without also optimizing its ability to collect the data it needs to do so. Reports, whether generated automatically by the EHR, created through custom coding or a third party, or compiled through tedious human work, can always be improved.

Optimization requires good data; good data require valid input. The most common error hospitals make when generating reports is to poorly define them. If I want to optimize decision making with regard to clinical alerts, for example, I need a report that gives me both valid and reliable data on this objective. In a report of why physicians override allergy alerts, if the data indicate that physicians always pick the top reason from the drop-down solely because clicking the top reason is faster, these data are stunningly reliable (physicians **always** pick this reason), but they are completely invalid (the top reason may or may not be the **actual** reason for over-riding the alert). We must define our reports so they measure what we actually need to know and do so validly **and** reliably.

In many cases, the most useful report gives us unexpected results, prompting action to identify the cause. For example, a simple report on the number of iatrogenic infections may identify a problem, even if the report wasn't aimed at identifying problems.

Many of the most important aspects of optimization involve "filing off the rough edges" of the orderables catalog, the order sets, or the modal order entry windows (MOEWs). This sort of optimization often relies on carefully defined, thoughtful reporting. If certain orderables are never ordered, can we delete an OEF (i.e., default the OEF in the background and ensure that the user doesn't have to see it) or make it optional, or can we edit the drop-down menu to include only appropriate options? If certain order sets are never used or contain orderables that are never checked, should they be deleted, renamed, or redesigned? Most order sets are—notwithstanding how much effort was put into their design—too long or don't accurately reflect real-world clinical care. A good report can identify the problem and point the way toward optimization. The same is true of MOEWs and department home folders: They can be created and improved, thereby speeding patient care and shaping best practice.

In any aspect of EHR usage—finding data, placing orders, or documenting—optimization is not a matter of having the most up-to-date versions or the "best" software as much as having the most user-friendly and efficient interfaces. To the user, the key features of optimization lie in decreasing the number of clicks, speeding the system's response to those clicks, ensuring system stability, decreasing extraneous information, and arranging the interfaces in a logical, intuitive format. Whether we are focused on orderables, order sets, MOEWs, documentation, data viewing, or alerts, the user needs to interact quickly, reliably, and intuitively. Optimization is a matter of making the EHR so user-friendly that it becomes all but "invisible" to the clinical user.

Optimization isn't the latest software, but the most usable software.

WORKFLOW OPTIMIZATION

Although much of the day-to-day aspects of clinical care—such as the nurses' report, physician rounds, and progress notes—remain unchanged from those of 50 years ago, there are notable changes in the details of our clinical workflows.

The long shelves of standard medical references that were common on hospital wards three decades ago have been replaced by electronic sources. Rather than merely look up arcane information, many of us regularly pull the latest information off the Internet, even for our standard cases. We routinely access information and

---

Optimization Goals

What should we optimize?

- Workflows
- Data acquisition
- Ordering process
- Clinical documentation
- Medical decision making
- Patient safety
- Clinical quality
- Billing process
- Regulatory compliance
- Hospital culture

---

brush up our understanding using evidence-based care, e-published journal articles, and specialty blogs. The speed with which we gather medical information has increased, the quality of that information has improved, and we are better able to locate the information we require to provide good care. Residents now continually recheck, validate, and update their medical knowledge as they practice. We do not just acquire new knowledge but also continuously tune our current knowledge.

Keeping Up with the Technology—and the Residents

A 30-minute discussion on updating hospital policy in regard to contacting consultants had been frustrating and confusing for many of the members of one hospital's physician advisory committee. While all agreed that personal contact needed to occur at some point, they were in total disagreement as to how the initial contact should be placed, variously arguing for a phone call by the unit secretary, a printed form hand-carried to the consultant, or an orderable sent to the consulting department, which would contact the attending physician consultant on call. In a lull in the argument, one of the committee members, a 50-year-old cardiologist, looked at his iPhone and began laughing. The other members asked him for an explanation, and he said:

"When I told the residents that I wouldn't be available this afternoon to respond to consultation requests, I was thinking of phone calls, and I assumed they wouldn't try to contact me. Frankly, it looks like all of our arguments are behind the times and that the residents are way ahead of us. They've automatically started sending all my consults to me by text message."

Overall workflows—ICU rounds, for example—have remained in place, but the way in which they are carried out is changing markedly. Residents now take at least one computer (often two, sometimes three) with them on their rounds. Access to patient information, placement of patient orders, and clinical documentation are generally faster and more efficient, even if the backbone of the workflow—for example, morning report when residents are gathered around an attending as they review their patient care—remains unchanged. Workflows may still be identifiably similar, but their efficiency and accuracy change.

Workflows are a key target for continual optimization. Many of the improvements to workflows have been technical: Residents quickly contact consultants via cell phone, e-mail, Vocera, or text messages without pausing to sit down. EKGs and radiology views are pulled up on a smartphone or tablet in the few seconds it takes to move between patient rooms. Orders are placed and underway long before rounds are finished. These changes can be disquieting—even anathema—to the older physician; residents are often the ones driving these changes.

DRIVING QUALITY MEDICAL CARE

Optimization is the ability to manage technical change while keeping a firm eye on the hospital's vision. Too often, policies simply are responses to technical change that give no thought to what those technical improvements might offer. For example, the use of electronic templates for documentation has obvious implications for improving our ability to document data and quickly access those data later. We can now generate an accurate report on how many of our CHF patients had a systolic blood pressure over 200 mmHg and how many of these patients received IV medications to lower the pressure during the past 12 months. While this capability is laudable and even useful, it does not speak to the real purpose of physicians' documentation: to convey the patient's story. While

I certainly want to know that the patient had CHF and which therapy was given, the key reason I access the physician documentation is to understand **why** the physician diagnosed CHF and **why** the physician chose that specific therapy. Physician documentation should never be a collection of data but a description of the physician's reasoning, his concerns, the way he weighed options, and his expectations. If a neurologist's documentation simply tells me the

---

The Key to Good Physician Documentation Isn't Facts; It's Perspective and Interpretation

Using an electronic template, an emergency physician was able to document a complete note, including all the technical details of the endotracheal intubation for the patient who had just arrived in the ICU. The emergency physician was pleased to see that—using macros—he had to click only twice to enter the intubation paragraph and that the remainder of his note was equally fast and efficient as well as up to standards for billing.

The intensivist who received the patient, however, was less impressed. The three-page note gave precise details regarding the patient's vital signs, initial physical findings, oxygenation, tube size, post-intubation X-ray findings, ventilator settings, and a host of other clinical data, but **nowhere in the note was there any indication of why the patient had been intubated or of the medical decision making that had occurred.** The intensivist said, "I end up ignoring the notes from this ED physician. His notes never tell me a single thing that I couldn't have gotten out of the computer myself. I still have no idea of what he was thinking. I always have to start my entire evaluation from scratch as though no other physician had been involved."

---

numbers for all of the patient's deep tendon reflexes and describes the patient's electroencephalogram, there is little value to the document; if it tells me that the patient had a stroke, explains how the neurologist arrived at this diagnosis, and then defines the patient's prognosis and suggested treatment, there is enormous value to the document. A physician's documentation is not data but experience, perspective, rational considerations, and actionable advice.

Physician documentation is not a compilation of data: It is an *explanation* of the data. If we simply adopt electronic templates and—through policy or neglect—allow physician documentation to become an efficient way to obtain mineable data, we are not optimizing patient care; we are undercutting it.

The same principle applies to all attempts at optimization. We must optimize the entire workflow with an eye toward improving patient care and not thoughtlessly optimize only the technical aspects of patient care. Improved technology can contribute to vastly better patient care, but improved technology is not—per se—the same as better care.

Optimization demands that we focus on quality, not technology.

KEY POINTS

- Optimization is both
  —the immediate tweaking that occurs post-conversion; and
  —an ongoing, permanent process critical to quality.
- Continual optimization has five aspects:
  —Adding EHR solutions
  —Updating the EHR
  —Keeping up to date with regulatory and financial requirements and recommendations
  —Keeping up to date with evidence-based standards
  —Optimizing clinical use of the EHR

- Optimizing clinical use is key:
  —New goals must be continually set.
  —Optimization depends on good data and reports.
  —Clinical workflows are a key target for optimization.
  —Quality must be optimized, not technology.
- Hospitals should optimize
  —workflows,
  —data acquisition,
  —the ordering process,
  —clinical documentation,
  —medical decision making,
  —patient safety,
  —clinical quality,
  —billing process,
  —regulatory compliance, and
  —hospital culture.

CHAPTER 12

Improving Medical Decisions

No matter what measures are taken, doctors will
sometimes falter, and it isn't reasonable
to ask that we achieve perfection.
What is reasonable is to ask
that we never cease to aim for it.

—Atul Gawande

WHILE EHRs DO not guarantee better care, they can help providers improve its quality and safety. This goal is laudable and consistent with effective EHR usage in general, but it also can be approached by intentionally building specific tools into EHRs. The most useful tools aim directly at the decision-making process.

Our understanding of human disease has grown, but our innate ability to comprehend its totality has not kept up. Until now, the answer has been to fracture medical care. Instead of ten diseases, we have ten thousand; instead of a general physician, we have ten specialists. Each specialist is an expert on a handful of problems; no physician can encompass the entirety of patient care. The typical hospital patient has an attending physician and multiple consultants, and the attending struggles to orchestrate a single useful plan from the esoteric advice of the consultants. This fracturing contributes to the problem of medical quality. It is difficult to bring all of current medical knowledge together into a coherent whole and equally difficult to bring all of our current clinical personnel—attending physicians, consultants, residents, radiologists, pharmacists, nurses, and myriad ancillary staff—together to ensure coherent, effective, and efficient patient care.

None of us has a perfect memory or unerring judgment, and we are generally unable to retain the breadth of medical knowledge, even within our own specialties. Hippocrates might have known all that was known then about medicine, but given our current body of medical knowledge, it is no longer feasible to keep abreast of the relevant medical literature, integrate all of the available patient data, and recall those data flawlessly in the midst of fatigue, stress,

---

Who's Treating My Patient?

In many hospitals, patients have not only multiple consultants but multiple attending physicians as well. Patients receiving academic hospitalist services in particular may have more than a dozen residents, multiple hospitalists (the attending physicians of record, who vary by shift and day of the week), and several consultants as well. Due to the large number of physicians who are responsible for coordinating a patient's care, care teams commonly are uncertain about which physician has placed which order.

During morning report, attending physicians commonly ask such questions as "Who ordered this CT scan?" or "Who put my patient on that antibiotic?" EHRs provide the answers to these questions; most display the name of the ordering physician for every order and are able to sort all orders by the name of the ordering physician.

Coordinating the totality of care still can be difficult (finding out **why** certain orders were placed can be especially challenging), but physicians can now be sure that they know **who** placed which orders.

---

and conflicting clinical demands. As a result, medical errors occur. The need to decrease those errors has prompted the burgeoning role of clinical decision support.

CLINICAL DECISION SUPPORT

Clinical decision support (CDS) is the use of electronic means to shape medical decisions and thereby improve the quality and safety of patient care. CDS also includes retrospective reporting (asynchronous support) to physicians and nurses on patient care they have already provided so they can make better decisions in the future. More critically, however, CDS provides real-time feedback and advice (synchronous support) to improve the decision process **as it occurs**. Synchronous CDS can prevent errors **before** they occur rather than simply report errors that have **already** occurred. In addition, CDS can even be used predictively to suggest appropriate medical actions before the physician would otherwise be aware of the need for intervention.

CDS is usually assumed to be beneficial, although its cost-effectiveness and actual medical benefit have been questioned and require careful consideration. Not all CDS is beneficial, and—to the contrary—**poorly designed** CDS can be detrimental to patient care, decreasing both quality and safety as well as increasing costs. As is true of EHRs in general, the benefit of CDS does not lie in the implementation itself but depends heavily on **how** CDS is designed and implemented.

What defines well-designed CDS and distinguishes it from poorly designed CDS? CDS is effective and beneficial only insofar as it

- fits into the clinical workflow efficiently and accurately;
- is synchronous (provided exactly at the moment a decision has to be [or should be] made);
- is not complex;

- provides clear, precise, relevant information to the decision maker; and
- does not impede or affect any other point in the clinical workflow.

Poorly designed CDS

- is asynchronous (provided after a medical decision has been made),
- fires frequently,
- is difficult to understand, and
- requires the user to make multiple clicks.

CDS Types

Most EHR vendors supply tools for CDS, and an increasing number of add-ons are also becoming commercially available from independent vendors. Moreover, the plethora of poorly designed CDS notwithstanding, the sophistication of CDS tools is rapidly improving. Decision support not only is available for clinical aspects of care but also is quickly coming to include financial aspects to ensure more efficient use of hospital resources, more accurate (and faster) billing, and prescriptions that are tailored to the patient's insurance coverage.

CDS supplied by EHR vendors runs a gamut, from simple allergy alerts to complex algorithms that help hospitals meet the requirements of meaningful use, quality benchmarks, and Joint Commission standards to a small but growing number of predictive algorithms that identify patient risks and head them off. Even the simplest alerts need to be carefully considered and customized, if only to exclude unnecessary pop-ups. The more complex and sophisticated the CDS, the more planning and care required to ensure the intended outcome and avoid unintended consequences.

Death by a Thousand Cuts

The CMIO of a hospital system in the Northeast believed that all alerts were valuable and that problems occurred only because users didn't have time to adapt to new alerts. He believed that there was no limit to the number of useful alerts as long as they were introduced piecemeal, so while he introduced only two alerts per month after conversion, he attempted to introduce all 115 standard vendor alerts over time.

Medical staff not only routinely bypassed the growing number of alerts but soon revolted as the number of alerts began to interfere with patient care. The CMIO quickly lost all political credibility—and then lost his position.

CDS quality is determined by excellence of design, not by quantity. Beyond the "native" CDS supplied by EHR vendors, other sources of CDS exist, including generic forms, such as references and links to order sets (usually supplied by vendors of such order sets), as well as independent add-on software intended solely for improving clinical decisions. Such software can be installed alongside the hospital EHR and can monitor all of a patient's data—such as a documented past medical history of myasthenia gravis—and provide dynamic alerting and suggestions for orders that might create patient risks, such as the use of magnesium sulfate during complications of preeclampsia in late pregnancy. Some of these programs not only respond instantly (synchronously) to any changes made to a patient's medical history (even if the ordering physician is completely unaware of the changes) but also suggest appropriate therapy based on patient weight, medications, and so forth. Similar programs provide therapeutic suggestions for appropriate antibiotics, based on allergies, previous antibiotic therapy, cultures, antibiotic resistance, fever, local patterns of drug sensitivity, and other clinical data. These and other independent, commercial CDS solutions offer much more than the simple alerts offered by most EHR vendors, and there is every reason to foster their development. Many of these solutions are designed by physicians and nurses, so the CDS is precisely tailored to the clinical problems they themselves face in actual practice. These specialized solutions—designed by clinicians—are a cottage industry of CDS applications, making these products quicker to respond to changing clinical needs than do those provided by some large EHR vendors and giving providers a wider choice of CDS tools.

There is a growing consensus that some aspects of CDS—particularly clinical data—should move "into the cloud." If a hospital has a single case of an unusual medical problem, it may go unidentified, but when clinical data are pooled on a county, state, national, or even global level, such problems become more apparent and therefore more amenable to solution. Some issues, such as drug side effects, viral epidemics, and prosthetic complications, are recognized only when national data are pooled. Not only can a large, national body of data contribute to the recognition of clinical risks; by using cloud-based approaches to CDS, we also can more rapidly institute the indicated changes in medical care. This approach has been taken by a major medical voice recognition service, which can identify a new medical term, such as the name of a new monoclonal antibody, within hours of its first use and then instantly update its ability to correctly recognize the new term when spoken by any user anywhere in the world. Cloud-computing CDS may enable faster recognition and response to epidemics or other rapidly changing medical problems, regardless of location.

In hospitals, CDS is changing from reactive support to predictive support. Software that uses complex algorithms to predict clinical events—such as solutions that monitor individual patient data (e.g., vital signs)—and patient risk (including cardiac arrest) is coming into general use. These solutions are being used to identify not only "pre-code" patients but also patients at risk of infection, falls, sepsis, and organ failure. Such CDS tools are becoming the de facto standard of care in many hospitals, and as their sophistication and reliability increases and they become mandated by regulation, they will likely become the *de jure* standard of care as well.

Truly dynamic CDS exists in certain add-on programs, but this approach has not yet been taken to its mature conclusion. Dynamic CDS changes (e.g., when it issues alerts, what it recommends, who it alerts) from moment to moment on the basis of changes made to patient data and documentation. This sophisticated tool is intended to provide finely tuned advice, changing drug, dose, and other recommendations on the basis of synchronous data. For example, when the nurse corrects errors in a patient's past medical history, when a new blood culture shows a specific pattern of resistance, or when unexpected oximetry values enter a chart, the pattern of advice changes and may even suggest that changes be made to previous orders.

Dynamic CDS aims to become transparent to the user, particularly as it becomes an integral part of the documentation process. For example, when a physician begins an admission note with documentation of "chest pain," it offers treatment plans and order sets consistent with a probable cardiac etiology. When the physician adds that the patient has "shortness of breath" and a "history of a blood coagulation disorder," the diagnostic and therapeutic suggestions dynamically change, becoming more consistent with the workup and treatment for a pulmonary embolus. It issues no alert and does not intrude on the user's experience; CDS becomes an organic part of the clinical workflow. Suggestions are continually adapted to the changing documentation and remain parallel to and supportive of the clinical decision-making workflow.

CDS Development

The CDS development process must support effective design. The question is not only **how** to design effective rules but also **which** rules (and how many) to develop. Moreover, CDS design is constrained by such factors as regulatory requirements, quality initiatives, and the financial needs of the hospital.

CDS oversight committees must have a long-term vision of what they want to accomplish as a hospital. The focus should not be catching errors but preventing them. Nuisance alerts slow patient care and do not promote optimal patient outcomes. Systematic, sophisticated management includes a well-defined charter that identifies specific improvement opportunities and goals, including

- designing CDS for specific targets,
- optimizing the acceptance and clinical value of CDS interventions, and
- measuring outcomes and altering CDS as necessary.

Not all rules should (or can) be implemented; build rules that address your hospital's critical needs. When choosing the order of priority, pick rules based on improving processes that your hospital has not done well. Evaluations done by The Joint Commission (where has the hospital been "dinged"?) and documentation of internal quality assurance, known risks, and medical errors will help you pinpoint these areas. Data gathered through *root cause analysis* (RCA), a process improvement tool used by many hospitals to evaluate medical errors, are invaluable not only for choosing which CDS rules to implement but also for designing **effective** CDS. Effective CDS directly targets the root causes of errors rather than their "symptoms" and is designed appropriately. **Investigating medical errors and learning from them are the keys to medical quality.**

Meaningful use, discussed earlier in this book, is a major external factor shaping CDS design. To achieve meaningful-use certification, hospitals' CDS rules must

- be authenticated by citing appropriate medical sources,
- be credible and based on clinical evidence,

- be sensitive to the patient context,
- invoke relevant medical knowledge,
- occur in a timely manner,
- be efficient in the workflow,
- integrate with the EHR, and
- be presented to the user who can take relevant action.

Additionally, an effective design process should allow rules to be discontinued or altered over time on the basis of changing clinical experience. Not only should rules change with changes in the formulary; rules that never fire, or that fire but never affect patient care, should be removed from the EHR. Rules are effective only if they change care for the better.

Any rule that doesn't improve patient care impedes patient care. Because all rules disrupt workflow to some extent, the value of any particular rule is always a balance between how much a rule **slows** patient care versus how often it **improves** patient care.

This observation raises a corollary: Whenever a new rule is built, it should be tried first in "silent mode" to see how often the rule would actually fire (assuming the rule is working as intended). If a rule never fires, fires too often, has no potential to change care, or doesn't match the intent of its design, delete the rule.

The most commonly identified error in the design process, however, is not simply the behavior of any particular rule but rather building too many rules, particularly if the rules seldom change medical decisions. This error—known as the "cry wolf problem"—causes alerts to fire so frequently that providers come to ignore or no longer notice them. ICU alerts—multiple auditory alarms from pumps, ventilators, and other medical equipment—commonly go unnoticed for this reason. **The more alerts you add, the less effective they become.**

In the design process, the practical rule of thumb is that for every new alert proposed, an existing alert should be deleted in exchange. This rule assumes that the current number of alerts is optimal and that fewer or more alerts would be counterproductive. Unfortunately, we don't know the optimal number of alerts, the optimal frequency of alerts, or how these theoretical optima might vary by user, location, or context.

The Case of the Disappearing Alerts

A national hospital chain had been using CPOE for several months, and the attending physicians in the ED had become inured to the multiple alerts that popped up regularly during delivery of patient care. In one 30-minute period, I observed a physician override six allergy alerts.

At the end of the period, I asked the physician if he had any problems with the recurrent allergy alerts. He looked puzzled and denied having seen any allergy alerts recently.

—Michael Fossel

If designing too many rules is the most common pitfall in CDS, then wishful thinking comes in a close second. A sophisticated approach to CDS involves having

1. a practical grasp of human nature and how users will actually respond, and
2. a detailed understanding of the problem you are attempting to solve.

If It's Too Hard, They'll Find a Way Around It

A community hospital in southern California developed a needlessly complex rule to ensure compliance with the guideline for thromboembolism prophylaxis. By the end of six months, data showed 100 percent compliance.

A careful look at the data, however, showed that the physicians had discovered that it took only a single click to document that "intervention was not medically indicated," while documenting the actual clinical therapy used for the patient required more than a dozen clicks and difficult navigation. Although patients were overwhelmingly given an appropriate intervention (e.g., an anticoagulation drug), the data showed that almost every patient had been documented as not needing an intervention.

Regardless of the actual care the physicians delivered (which was generally appropriate but well might not have been), the CDS made accurate documentation confusing, disrupted workflow, and slowed patient care. Physicians had simply found a way to avoid doing "extra work."

The error lay not with lazy physicians but with lazy CDS design.

Absent these two requirements, unintended consequences and ineffectual outcomes will result. Regarding the first factor—human nature—there is an unfortunate tendency to blame failed CDS on users who are pejoratively characterized as lazy or disruptive. The reality is that correctly designed CDS encourages good clinical behavior, and, conversely, poor clinical behavior almost always results from poor CDS design. The way to get clinical personnel to wash their hands is to make it easy to do so, not to rail against their "lazy" failure to find the hidden sink. Regarding the second factor, it is important to target the underlying problem (e.g., identified through RCA) rather than the superficial result. In medicine, we need to treat an underlying infection rather than simply cover up the associated fever; in CDS design, we need to prevent the underlying error rather than simply cover up the outcome of that error.

In addition to having all the characteristics discussed thus far, good design addresses six critical questions: *what, who, how, where, when*, and *why*. If a CDS rule fails to correctly answer these questions, it will interfere with provider workflow and—in the long run—decrease the quality of patient care. The "why" is the objective of the CDS rule itself, so let's turn our attention to the other five questions.

What *Information Should Be Delivered in a CDS Alert?*

Information must be sculpted to exclude extraneous information and include the critical data physicians need to make a correct medical decision. A CDS alert regarding a potential drug interaction, for example, should not include information on extraneous labs, nor should it include dosage, side effects, route, or other drug information unless such information is crucial to the decision. Extraneous information is white noise that confuses and exasperates the user and delays the delivery of care. In some cases, an entire alert may be white noise, such as one that fires when a typical side effect of a medication (e.g., itching in response to opioids) is mistakenly listed as an allergy.

Who *Should Receive the CDS Alert?*

CDS rules should target providers who are able to change their current orders and are medically responsible for their patients. Specifically, alerts should appear to providers who have CPOE privileges and can be expected to assume responsibility for care. Alerts have no value if they fire to users who cannot (or cannot be expected to) take action.

If, for example, a patient has been on amoxicillin for the past two weeks, stops the medication at the time of hospital admission, and gives the triage nurse a history of a "penicillin allergy," this information will trigger a "reverse allergy checking" alert to the nurse. Even

> ### Reverse Allergy Checking
>
> *Reverse allergy checking* is a type of asynchronous alert that
> fires, for example, when a nurse enters a history of an
> allergy to a medication the patient already has been given.
> While it may be beneficial to the attending physician, it is
> of little value to the pharmacy staff or nurse. Pharmacists
> and nurses aren't able to proactively respond to the
> alert; they can be only reactive, calling a provider to see
> if the patient has already had a reaction to the previously
> prescribed medication or if the provider actually meant to
> prescribe the drug to which the patient is now known to be
> allergic. Similarly, reverse allergy checking will fire for home
> meds that may not have been converted to inpatient meds,
> and the pharmacy will receive a misleading alert. Moreover,
> the pharmacist or nurse may have no idea why a drug was
> prescribed or whether the reverse allergy alert should be
> overridden.

though the nurse observes no allergic reaction to the amoxicillin,
she should not be expected to delete the history of penicillin allergy
that prompted the alert. Such an alert might be beneficial to the
admitting physician as he does the patient's admission medication
reconciliation, but it is of little value to the triage nurse. If an alert
goes to the wrong person, that person has to call the provider it
should have gone to, and care is delayed.

Every CDS rule should target a specific role, and alerts should
not appear unnecessarily.

How *Should the Information Be Presented?*
CDS alerts should be concise, offering clear options that require
minimal action. Some drug–drug interaction alerts, for example,
require that the user click on each of the interacting drugs and
drill down to find the concern and therapeutic options. Such alerts

should convey the information that the provider needs to make a clinical prescribing decision immediately on the initial screen, not require the provider to click or scroll. The alert should succinctly and clearly state the next action that the provider should take and then offer options that can be executed with a single click. In the case of canceling, changing, or overriding a drug–drug interaction, the screen should summarize the concern and then offer three

---

How to Use CDS to Increase Risk, Slow Patient Care, and Annoy Users

A Florida hospital had a CDS alert that fired to ensure that every patient with a potential myocardial infarction was given aspirin or that an acceptable reason was given for not giving the aspirin. The initial screen showed only the regulation and required that the user click to see suggested responses. This next view included widely spaced options that filled three screens and hence required users to scroll to view all of them. The most common option—that aspirin had been given—not only was the very last option on the last screen but also wasn't identified by the system so that the CDS wouldn't fire in the first place. Moreover, if users chose to order the aspirin while viewing the CDS screens, they could not do so in a single click; they had to exit the screens, find the order screen, and search for the drug and the correct dose. Finally, users were required to sign the last screen electronically to confirm that they were aware of their responsibility to give aspirin to all patients with a potential myocardial infarction.

Another hospital, also in Florida, had a single-screen CDS alert for this same function. It fired only **if** aspirin had not been given and then only **if** an aspirin allergy had not been documented. It offered users three options, each of which could be selected with a single click.

---

options: a single click to cancel the order, a single click to order an alternative medication, and a single click to override the interaction warning and continue with the original order.

CDS alerts that involve multiple screens, are difficult to interpret, or feature a drop-down menu of choices—particularly lengthy drop-downs that the provider must scroll through—need to be redesigned. The format should be unambiguous, simple, and easy to navigate.

Where *Should CDS Be Delivered?*

An EHR can provide decision support in a number of different ways. Alerts are only one of such methods and seldom the most effective or efficient. The best alerts are those that never fire because there is a more efficient way of accomplishing their intention. Some EHRs, for example, fire an alert when a physician orders an expensive antibiotic, suggesting a less expensive alternative on the formulary. The incidence of this alert goes down, however, when the order sets and MOEWs offer the more acceptable alternative. In this case, physicians tend to choose the cheaper alternative because (1) it's already an option in the order set they were going to select, (2) it can be ordered with a single click via the MOEW, and (3) the more expensive antibiotic has to be typed into the OEF. In short,

---

Modifying CDS to Ensure Ease of Use

A hospital in the Southwest had an alert that fired whenever a physician ordered certain antibiotics by IV, suggesting oral alternatives. Taking this suggestion required that the physician back out of the order, search for the alternate drug, and place the new order. Building these preferred routes into the standard order sets and placing them on the MOEWs markedly reduced the frequency of the alert, and the physicians found the new system less intrusive and more efficient.

---

users prefer the cheaper antibiotic because it is easier to order; the system's built-in CDS addresses the issue up front, and the alert is not triggered.

CDS should always encourage providers to choose the channel that poses the least impediment to care and produces the best results. In a perfect world, EHRs would be so well designed that users would almost never see alerts or pop-ups. If the required (and preferably defaulted) OEFs for an antibiotic show a stop date consistent with accepted usage, physicians rarely will order continual antibiotics or see alerts warning them that a course of antibiotics should not exceed the given duration.

When *Should CDS Be Provided?*

Well-designed CDS delivers advice at the precise moment a medical decision is made. While there is occasionally value in

---

Not "The Error You Made Yesterday" but "How to Deliver the Best Care Right Now"

A small community hospital had a problem meeting the requirement that blood cultures be drawn **before** antibiotics are given to patients admitted for pneumonia. The alert triggered whenever blood cultures were ordered for a newly admitted patient who had a recent order for antibiotics. In effect, the alert informed physicians that they had already made an error, had no effect on the rate of regulatory compliance, and annoyed users because there was no action they could take to correct the error.

The alert was redesigned to fire whenever antibiotics were ordered for newly admitted pneumonia patients. It explained the requirement in one sentence and then offered a single-click option to order two blood cultures.

The hospital immediately achieved regulatory compliance.

---

providing guidance **prior** to a decision point, users may forget the guidance if it is given too early. When information is given too late, users have to redo their work and thus are more likely to ignore the guidance to avoid that extra work. Any other timing not only is inefficient but also tends to impede rather than improve the quality of decision making and the overall workflow.

Prompting Medical Actions

CDS has a broader role than simply catching errors at the time a decision is made: It must prompt actions that the physician is yet unaware of. In this case, CDS is triggered by events that might not have come to the attention of the physician or nurse but must be decided and acted on. The most common example is a laboratory

---

Locking the Barn Door After the Horse Escaped (or died)

A recent national case involved the death of a boy who presented at an ED with clinical evidence of infection. The white-cell count was unexpectedly high, but the result came back after the boy was discharged and was not brought to the attention of his physicians.

This exact scenario has occurred—in one form or another—in most hospitals. Similarly, many hospitals have been able to "retrospectively predict" patient problems, but while the clinical data were present before complications occurred, there was no effective way of alerting the clinical staff.

In all of these cases, it was retrospectively clear that the patient would have problems, but prospectively no one was ever made aware of the dangers. Many suggest that CDS could be used to prevent such complications and deaths.

---

result, such as high potassium or a positive blood culture. In many hospitals, such results are routinely brought to the attention of the clinical staff, but with the advent of CDS we may be able to ensure a greater degree of reliability that the information is not only communicated but acted on. In the case of high potassium, for example, the alert may include the usual options for treating hyperkalemia, complete with doses tailored to weight and actionable with a single click. This approach may not only increase the likelihood that physicians' response will be medically appropriate but also markedly decrease both the time to delivery of effective care and the potential for calculation errors.

CONCLUSIONS

We are in the midst of a shift from care led by a single physician to care not only provided by a team but also directed as a team activity. It is clear that physicians—whether they be surgeons, hospitalists, or emergency physicians—are gradually becoming part of this team. Surgeons no longer make decisions by fiat, nor is tyrannical behavior tolerated. Hospitalists and emergency physicians are used to working with nurses and other patient care workers throughout the delivery of care. Nurses do not "own" patient care, and neither do physicians. Step by step we are evolving into a culture of patient care in which we have a shared responsibility for quality. We have come to accept input from the quality review worker, the infectious disease nurse, the social worker, the nutritional consultant, and all other members of the team who contribute to better patient care. Physicians' leadership is valuable not because they are physicians but because they contribute value to this broader, shared view of patient care. The intensely specific knowledge of consultants—or of any narrow approach to medicine—is of little value unless it aligns with the totality of patient care.

The same question of who's running the show is playing out in medical IT. A decade ago, computers in medicine were often the territory of IT departments; IT staff decided what to buy and how to implement what they bought, and they defined the goals of IT projects. Curiously, the hospitals that were led by IT were most likely to fail.

EHRs cannot—and will never—lead the patient care team. The most that software can do is provide a framework: reminders, an overall plan of care, a safety net, and a way of keeping track of the otherwise marginally coordinated members of the clinical team.

Quality improvement is continual; the use of EHRs as a quality improvement tool is no different. The degree to which medical software can help providers improve patient care will accrue gradually; improvement is not a onetime event. While conversion to an EHR does not guarantee quality clinical care, it is the beginning—not the end—of a quality improvement process.

Our clinical workflow and technology are transitioning simultaneously. The technology will continue to improve, and it promises to support, rather than threaten, the heart of good medical care. But we cannot afford to lose sight of the reason that drives technical improvements. People do not go into medicine because they feel driven to meet regulatory burdens or use computers. Nurses do not enter the profession so that they can click boxes with a mouse.

The end goal is not better technology but better patient care.

KEY POINTS

- Well-designed CDS
  —fits into the clinical workflow;
  —is provided when support is useful;
  —is clear, precise, and relevant; and
  —does not cry wolf.
- The design process for CDS should
  —identify specific goals,
  —target specific roles,
  —encourage acceptance and optimize clinical value, and
  —measure outcomes and alter CDS in response if necessary.

- Effective CDS design depends on six key questions:
  —Why should CDS be provided?
  —What information should be presented?
  —Who should receive it?
  —How should it be presented?
  —Where should it be provided?
  —When should it be delivered?

Glossary

ADE: Adverse drug event.

Alert: A warning displayed to users, advising them of risk or providing significant information. Alerts may be overridden and require that the user enter additional information (e.g., the reason for the override) or perform additional actions.

AMI: Acute myocardial infarction; one of the core measures issued by The Joint Commission and CMS.

ANES: Abbreviation for anesthesia or anesthesiology, commonly used in order set nomenclature.

American Recovery and Reinvestment Act of 2009 (ARRA): Legislation mandating the use of medical IT in American hospitals, commonly called the "stimulus" or "recovery" act. See *meaningful use*.

Asynchronous support: CDS that is provided after a medical decision has been made. Compare to *synchronous support*.

Autotext: A macro function in some electronic documentation.

Backfilling: Finding staff to fill positions temporarily left empty, usually during training.

Big bang: Conversion of the whole hospital to a solution (e.g., to CPOE) or conversion of a specific unit of the hospital to multiple solutions (e.g., CPOE and documentation). See also the antonym *sequential conversion*.

Build: The version of the vendor software being developed for release to clinical users.

CAC: Children's asthma care; one of the core measures issued by The Joint Commission and CMS.

Catalog: A complete list of all possible items or actions that can be ordered in a hospital.

CBC: Complete blood count; includes red- and white-cell counts as well as other data.

CDS: Clinical decision support. See *decision support*.

Change control: The process by which domain changes (e.g., modification of orderables, privileges, functions, and settings) are managed in the post-conversion phase.

CHF: Congestive heart failure.

CIO: Chief information officer.

Circle-back training: The process of returning to reevaluate and retrain users after an initial period of EHR use, usually to fine-tune skills and customize filters and settings to achieve greater proficiency and efficiency.

Cloud: Nonlocalized data storage accessible via the Internet, as opposed to data storage in a local hospital computer.

CME: Continuing medical education.

CMIO: Chief medical information officer.

CMO: Chief medical officer.

CMS: Centers for Medicare & Medicaid Services; the federal agency that administers Medicare, Medicaid, and the Children's Health Insurance Program.

CNO: Chief nursing officer.

Command center: The location of staff managing the conversion, typically analysts, super-users, and those involved in program governance, as well as change control (q.v.).

Communication order: An order primarily intended to communicate information; generally does not request a medication, laboratory test, radiology exam, or other similar orderable.

Compliance: The degree to which clinical personnel actually use an EHR or, with regard to regulatory standards, the degree to which the hospital is able to meet such requirements (e.g., meaningful use, q.v.).

Condition: In the context of this book, the status of a patient's medical state (e.g., acute, chronic, stable).

Convenience order set: An order set made up of similar types of orders (e.g., an antibiotics order set, a laboratory tests order set, a pain medications order set), not organized by clinical pathway (e.g., an admission for myocardial infarction order set).

Conventions: Hospital-wide agreements as to how orderables or order sets should be named.

Conversion: The phase of implementation in which users begin to use the EHR for patient care, typically the day the EHR is turned on as well as the following several days. See also *go-live*.

COWs: Computers on wheels; computers that can be wheeled through a clinical unit. See also *WOWs*.

CPOE: Computerized physician (or provider) order entry.

Cry wolf: Alerts that fire so frequently that the user habituates to them and ultimately comes to ignore them, thereby increasing patient risk.

C-suite: The generic term for hospital administrators at the executive level, typically the CEO, COO, CIO, CMO, CNO, and so forth.

CT scan: Computed tomography scan.

Decision support: A software solution that can advise or guide medical care, especially at the time a clinical decision is being made.

Default: The use of the most common value to prefill an option, for example, a dose of 1 gm for Ancef.

Departmental home folder: The initial screen that users see when they place orders, usually defined for their specialty (e.g., orthopedic departmental home folder); often used synonymously with *MOEW* (q.v.).

Devices: The hardware components of EHR use, typically desktops, laptops, tablets, smartphones, wireless technology, and display screens.

Ding: An informal verb referring to citations from The Joint Commission with regard to hospital problems or perceived risks.

Durable medical equipment (DME): Orderables such as crutches and home oxygen, often ordered for home use.

Door-to-doctor time: The time that elapses between the moment the patient enters a facility (e.g., the emergency department) and the time the patient is seen by a physician.

Doppler: An ultrasound study that evaluates blood flow.

Dose range checking: A feature that compares the ordered dose to standard dose limits, often on the basis of dose per unit weight; especially useful for pediatric and oncology patients.

Downtime: A period during which the EHR is unavailable either for planned (e.g., upgrades) or unplanned (e.g., computer crash) reasons.

DRG: Diagnosis-Related Group; a categorization of diagnoses, largely derived from billing (rather than clinical) concerns.

Dual-tasking orders: A single order that actually places two (or more) orders. See *linked orders*.

Duplicate checking: A feature that informs the user that a duplicate action is occurring (e.g., two similar drug orders, two identical laboratory tests). The duplicate actions usually must occur within a defined time window to trigger this check (e.g., two identical laboratory orders within a 24-hour period).

Dynamic CDS: A decision support feature that alters documentation templates, options, differential diagnoses, suggested clinical actions, available orders, and other aspects of the EHR interface on a moment-to-moment basis as a result of any change in real-time clinical data.

ED: Emergency department.

ED throughput: The ability of an emergency department to efficiency and quickly treat patients.

EHR: Electronic health record; often used interchangeably with EMR (electronic medical record). The term *EHR* typically is used in a broader sense to encompass the entire system rather than merely the patient record. The term *EMR* typically is used in a more restrictive sense to include only the patient record rather than the entire system.

EP: In the context of this book, *EP* refers to eligible professionals, who have defined requirements under meaningful use (q.v.).

Epi: Epinephrine (adrenaline).

e-publish: To publish electronically (as opposed to on paper).

Favorite folders: Collections of orderables (or diagnoses or other items) that have been saved by an individual user into personal folders so the user can easily retrieve those items in the future. See also *home folders*.

Formulary: A catalog of drugs, either national, within a hospital, or for a pharmacy.

Formulary mismatch: The inability to match formulary items during medication reconciliation.

Geographic phases: An approach to conversion in which certain units (e.g., the ED) convert, later followed by other units (e.g., all inpatient units). Compare to *sequential conversion*.

Go-live: The phase of implementation in which users begin to use the EHR for patient care, typically the day the EHR is turned on as well as the following several days. See also *conversion*.

Governance: The political structure that is responsible for decisions and actions in a hospital.

GYN: Gynecology.

HF: Heart failure; one of the core measures issued by The Joint Commission and CMS. See also *CHF*.

Health Insurance Portability and Accountability Act (HIPAA): Legislation that defines and requires a plethora of hospital and clinical actions, especially in regard to confidentiality, system security, and certain rights to healthcare access.

Home folders: Collections of orderables that have been saved by a department or specialty into folders so they may be easily retrieved in the future. See also *favorite folders*.

If-then orders: A primary order that triggers a secondary order under specified circumstances. Secondary orders necessitated by the entry of a primary order are also referred to as *hidden orders*. For example, the provider might order a CBC, specifying that a second order for a reticulocyte count should be entered if the hemoglobin result (from the CBC) is less than some value.

Implementation: The process of converting to a medical software product, typically a period of several months or more from initial plan to conversion.

Interaction checking: A feature that compares two (or more) drugs and alerts the provider to potential interactions.

Interface: The part of the computer—including but not limited to the visual elements displayed on a computer screen—that the user sees and interacts with.

IT: Information technology.

Joint Commission: A private organization that evaluates and regulates healthcare organizations.

Kitchen-sink order set: An order set that includes too many orders and therefore is difficult to use and slows patient care.

Layered macros: Multiple macros—at several levels—used to progressively hone in on specific findings, enabling physicians to document a much larger range of findings than would otherwise be possible.

Linked orders: Two or more orders that need to be ordered and completed in coordination.

LOS: Length of stay; the total time a patient stays either in a hospital or on a specific unit (e.g., the ED).

Macro: A way of setting a single click to perform several functions simultaneously.

Meaningful use: A series of governmental regulations intended to promote practical and effective use of EHRs to improve patient care.

Med-surg: Medical-surgical; usually refers to hospital wards with a mixed patient population.

Meds rec: Medication reconciliation; updating and correcting the list of a patient's medications. Usually divided into three types: admission meds rec, transfer meds rec, and discharge meds rec.

MOEW: Modal order entry window; the initial screen that users see when they place orders. Often used synonymously with departmental home folder (q.v.).

MRI: Magnetic resonance imaging.

Multum: A proprietary drug database with dynamic functions, often used in conjunction with EHRs.

Naming conventions: The rules for naming orderables and order sets, also referred to as *nomenclature rules*.

Niche system: An EHR that functions only within a specific area of the hospital (e.g., the ED).

Nomenclature: A system for naming orderables and order sets. See also *naming conventions*.

NPO: Nothing by mouth (derived from the Latin phrase *nil per os*).

NSAID: Non-steroidal anti-inflammatory drug; examples include ibuprofen and ketorolac.

OEF: Order entry field; specifies the details of an order, such as dose, route, frequency, and reason for exam.

Optimization: The phase of EHR usage during which the system (hardware, software, and especially workflow) is tweaked to maximize ease of use, safety, and response time.

Order set: A collection of orders that can be placed together as a single unit.

Orderable: Any item that can be ordered from the hospital catalog.

Ortho: Orthopedics.

PAC: Physician advisory committee. See also *PAG*.

PACS: Picture archiving and communication system; a system that allows users to see and interact with radiology images in a computer database.

PACU: Post-anesthesia care unit.

PAG: Physician advisory group. See also *PAC*.

Partial conversion: A conversion in which certain processes (e.g., documentation during medical codes) are left on paper.

Parallel ordering: The process of placing multiple orders simultaneously so that they are carried out in parallel. Compare to *serial ordering*.

Partial meds rec: A medication reconciliation that is incomplete, often performed when more than one physician is caring for a particular patient. One physician may perform a partial meds rec, and then the second physician will complete the meds rec.

PCA: Patient-controlled analgesia; typically an IV of an opiate that is self-administered by the patient (within preset dosage limits).

Peds: Pediatrics.

PNE: Pneumonia; one of the core measures issued by The Joint Commission and CMS.

PO: Oral.

Point-of-care (POC) tests: Clinical laboratory tests, such as blood glucose, that are processed on the ward (or in the ED, for example) rather than sent to the laboratory.

PowerPlan: A special type of order set created by Cerner Corporation.

PR: Pregnancy and related conditions; one of the core measures issued by The Joint Commission and CMS.

Pre-checked order: An order, usually within an order set, that is defaulted so that if the order set is signed, the order will become active. See also *unchecked order*.

Press Ganey: An independent corporation that ranks hospitals and other healthcare delivery systems.

Primary term: The main name for an orderable, as opposed to various synonyms. See also *secondary term*.

Privileges: The functions that a specific user has access to within a domain.

Procedure macros: The use of macros to document a range of specific procedures, such as joint reductions, intubations, and simple surgical procedures.

Provider: In medical IT, users who have privileges to place CPOE orders (e.g., physicians, midlevel practitioners, residents).

Protocol orders: Orders that are defined by a formal (usually written) hospital protocol.

qd: Daily.

RCA: Root cause analysis; the process of identifying the underlying cause of a problem rather than addressing the superficial symptoms of a problem.

RFE: Reason for exam; the clinical rationale for a particular test (e.g., chest pain, rapid heart rate), generally a radiology procedure.

RHO: Remote hosted organization; an organization whose computer database is managed by an outside contractor.

SCIP: Surgical Care Improvement Project.

Scope-of-practice orders: Orders that are considered within the scope of practice (usually nursing) and generally do not require a physician signature.

Scribe: A person who acts for a physician. Scribes may document for the physician or (more rarely) help place orders, but they have no direct clinical responsibilities.

Secondary term: Any of various synonyms for an orderable, as opposed to the primary term (q.v.).

Sequential conversion: A conversion in which either a hospital converts unit by unit (e.g., to CPOE) or a specific unit converts to several solutions one by one (e.g., to CPOE and documentation). See also the antonym *big bang*.

Serial ordering: The process of placing multiple orders one at a time, thereby delaying order completion and slowing patient care. Compare to *parallel ordering*.

Source: When used as an OEF, the origin of a lab sample (e.g., blood, urine, sputum).

Standing orders: Protocol orders that have been formally defined and instituted by the hospital for specific circumstances (e.g., codes, low blood sugar, IV site care). Protocol orders usually must be signed by a physician.

STK: Stroke; one of the core measures issued by The Joint Commission and CMS.

Super-user: A designated user with extra training who is responsible for helping others during implementation.

Synchronous support: CDS that occurs exactly at the moment a decision is being (or should be) made. Compare to *asynchronous support*.

TAT: Turnaround time. This term often is used in reference to lab results, operating room availability, and other measures of clinical efficiency.

Three Ps: Privileges, passwords, and printers; the most common sources of user problems on the first day of conversion.

TNF: Template non-formulary; a drug order for a medication not currently found in the formulary (e.g., an order for a recently released medication or a compound medication that is not yet listed).

Total parenteral nutrition (TPN): A complex set of orders encompassing all additives needed to provide parenteral nutrition.

Triage orders: Also called ATP (advanced triage protocol) orders. A set of orders, usually in the ED, intended for use by the nursing staff to begin prompt and efficient medical care before a physician examines the patient. Triage orders are generally formal, institutionally defined protocols.

Unchecked order: An order, usually within an order set, that is defaulted in an unchecked state so that it must be checked to be activated when the order set is signed. See also *pre-checked order*.

Unclean medications history: A medications history that is, for whatever reason, inaccurate.

Vag: Vaginal.

Vendors: Commercial sources of EHRs.

Virtual bed: A temporary bed, often in the ED, that holds a patient while he/she is waiting for an inpatient bed in the hospital.

Virtualized: As in *virtualized orderables*: orderables that may be seen and ordered by one user (or in one hospital) but not by another user (or in another hospital).

VTE: Venous thromboembolism; one of the core measures issued by The Joint Commission and CMS.

Web-based training (WBT): Use of the Internet (or software) to deliver training. WBT typically is less costly, but often less effective, than classroom-based training.

Wet read: The initial reading of a radiology examination, which later may be altered or amended.

Workflow: The sequence of clinical actions that define the work of physicians, nurses, and other clinical personnel.

WOWs: Workstations on wheels; a computer that can be wheeled through a clinical unit. See also *COWs*.

Resources

With so much information now online,
it is exceptionally easy to simply dive in and drown.

—*Alfred Glossbrenner*

WHEN IT COMES to EHRs, it seems that everyone is an expert—particularly if you do what most people do: Google the term! With 45.4 million hits for "electronic health record," you would have to do a lot of reading to make sense of it all.

When it comes to making decisions about system selection and implementation, understanding meaningful use, defining best practices, or uncovering shared lessons from other organizations, access to trusted, unbiased information is always helpful.

In our research for this book and in our everyday work, we've come across valuable information, and we want to share it with you to help you as you embark or continue on your EHR journey.

USEFUL WEBSITES

American College of Healthcare Executives (ACHE)
(www.ache.org)

ACHE is an international professional society of more than 40,000 executives who lead hospitals, healthcare systems, and other healthcare organizations. ACHE is a great resource for webinars, books, local chapter dinner meetings, and Level 1 accredited sessions specifically dedicated to EHR adoption and meaningful use.

Black Book Rankings (www.blackbookrankings.com/healthcare)

A market research company founded in 2002, Black Book Rankings provides rankings and for-fee detailed reports on top hospital and physician EHR systems as well as on other areas related to healthcare.

Health IT Home, US Department of Health & Human Services (http://healthit.hhs.gov)

This site offers a wealth of US government–provided resources specifically dedicated to health IT, EHRs, meaningful use, certification, HITECH programs, and more.

Healthcare Information and Management Systems Society (HIMSS) (www.himss.org)

HIMSS, a not-for-profit organization of more than 44,000 members, is focused on providing global leadership for the optimal use of IT and management systems for the betterment of healthcare. This site offers the latest information, reports, and live meetings dedicated to EHR adoption, best practices, and meaningful use.

HIMSS Analytics (www.himssanalytics.org)

HIMSS Analytics supports improved decision making for healthcare organizations, healthcare IT companies, and consulting firms by providing access to high-quality reports, data, and analytical expertise.

HELPFUL ARTICLES

Amarasingham, R., L. Plantinga, M. Diener-West, D. J. Gaskin, and N. R. Powe. 2009. "Clinical Information Technologies and Inpatient Outcomes: A Multiple Hospital Study." *Archives of Internal Medicine* 169 (2): 108–14. http://archinte .jamanetwork.com/article.aspx?articleid=414740.

American Hospital Association. 2011. "Hospitals and Care Systems of the Future." AHA Committee on Performance Improvement. www.aha.org/content/11/ hospitals-care-systems-of-future.pdf.

American Medical Association. 2011. "15 Questions to Ask Before Signing an EMR/ EHR Agreement." www.ama-assn.org/resources/doc/hit/emragreement.pdf.

Congressional Budget Office. 2008. "Evidence on the Costs and Benefits of Health Information Technology." www.cbo.gov/sites/default/files/cbofiles/ ftpdocs/91xx/doc9168/05-20-healthit.pdf.

Conn, J. 2010. "Docs Weigh in on Use of Scribes in Primary Care." ModernHealthcare.com. www.modernhealthcare.com/article/20100209/ NEWS/302099984.

DesRoches, C. M., E. G. Campbell, S. R. Rao, K. Donelan, T. G. Ferris, A. Jha, R. Kaushal, D. E. Levy, S. Rosenbaum, A. E. Shields, and D. Blumenthal. 2008. "Electronic Health Records in Ambulatory Care—A National Survey of Physicians." *New England Journal of Medicine* 359 (1): 50–60. www.nejm.org/doi/full/10.1056/ NEJMsa0802005#t=articleTop.

Edsall, R. L., and K. G. Adler. 2008. "User Satisfaction with EHRs: Report of a Survey of 422 Family Physicians." *Family Practice Management* 15 (2): 25–32. www.aafp.org/fpm/2008/0200/p25.html.

Frankovich, J., C. A. Longhurst, and S. M. Sutherland. 2011. "Evidence-Based Medicine in the EMR Era." *New England Journal of Medicine* 365: 1758–59. www.nejm.org/doi/full/10.1056/NEJMp1108726.

Mangalmurti, S. S., L. Murtagh, and M. M. Mello. 2010. "Medical Malpractice Liability in the Age of Electronic Health Records." *New England Journal of Medicine* 363 (21): 2060–67. www.nejm.org/doi/pdf/10.1056/NEJMhle1005210.

Mekhjian, H. S., R. R. Kumar, L. Kuehn, T. D. Bentley, P. Teater, A. Thomas, B. Payne, and A. Ahmad. 2002. "Immediate Benefits Realized Following Implementation of Physician Order Entry at an Academic Medical Center." *Journal of the American Medical Informatics Association* 9 (5): 529–39. www.ncbi.nlm.nih.gov/pmc/articles/PMC346640.

References

Advisory Board Company and HIMSS Analytics. 2012. "EMR Benefits and Benefit Realization Methods of Stage 6 and 7 Hospitals." Published in February. www.himssanalytics.org/research/AssetDetail.aspx?pubid=79509&tid=122.

Black Book Rankings. 2012. "2012 Rankings—Inpatient EHR Systems." www.blackbookrankings.com/healthcare/rankings-inpatient-ehr-systems.php.

Cebul, R. D., T. E. Love, A. K. Jain, and C. J. Hebert. 2011. "Electronic Health Records and Quality of Diabetes Care." *New England Journal of Medicine* 365 (9): 825–33.

Centers for Medicare & Medicaid Services (CMS). 2012. "Eligible Hospital and CAH Meaningful Use Table of Contents Core and Menu Set Objectives." www.cms.gov/Regulations-and-Guidance/Legislation/EHRIncentivePrograms/downloads/Hosp_CAH_MU-TOC.pdf.

Flexner, A. 1910. *Medical Education in the United States and Canada: A Report to the Carnegie Foundation for the Advancement of Teaching.* Boston: Merrymount Press.

Frankovich, J., C. A. Longhurst, and S. M. Sutherland. 2011. "Evidence-Based Medicine in the EMR Era." *New England Journal of Medicine* 365 (19): 1758–59.

Heifetz, R. A. 1998. *Leadership Without Easy Answers.* Cambridge, MA: Harvard University Press.

Institute of Medicine (IOM). 1999. *To Err Is Human.* Washington, DC: National Academies Press.

Lorenzi, N. M., A. Kouroubali, D. E. Detmer, and M. Bloomrosen. 2009. "How to Successfully Select and Implement Electronic Health Records (EHR) in Small Ambulatory Practice Settings." *BMC Medical Informatics and Decision Making* (February 23). www.biomedcentral.com/1472-6947/9/15.

National Guideline Clearinghouse. 2012. "Guideline Summary: Venous Thromboembolism Prophylaxis." Agency for Healthcare Research and Quality. http://guideline.gov/content.aspx?id=34841.

Sweeney, J. F. 2012. "Most Hospital Errors Not Reported." *Medical Economics* (February 25). www.modernmedicine.com/modernmedicine/Modern+Medicine +Now/Most-hospital-errors-not-reported/ArticleStandard/Article/detail/758988.

US Department of Health & Human Services (HHS). 2012. "HHS Secretary Kathleen Sebelius Announces Major Progress in Doctors, Hospital Use of Health Information Technology." News release, February 17. www.hhs.gov/news/press/ 2012pres/02/20120217a.html.

Index

BMJ Group, 96, 98

Budgeting/budgets, for electronic health record systems: for hardware and devices, 190; for training, 159

Buffet, Warren, 119

Burnout, among electronic health record system trainers, 164

Cardiologists, order sets of, 114

Care sets, 89. *See also* Order sets

Catalogs, computerized: categories of, 72; "cleaning up" of, 72–73; costs of, 77–78; definition of, 71, 268; issues regarding protocols and informal orders, 79–81; local, 71–72; medical issues, 84–86; multiple, 78–82; policy issues, 77–78; special issues, 83; "up-front" and "back-end," 79. *See also* Orderables

Centers for Medicare & Medicaid Services (CMS): core measures requirements of, 186–187; electronic health record system requirements of, 35; meaningful-use requirements of. *See* Meaningful-use requirements

Cerner, 27, 37–38, 39, 98; PowerPlan order sets from, 89, 101, 117, 275

Certification: of hospitals, 168; of vendors, 176

Change control, 220–224; definition of, 268; executive summaries in, 223–224

Charisma, of leaders, 44

Charts: medication, 65; simultaneous use of, 64–65

Chenault, Kenneth, 43

Chest x-ray orders: orderable nomenclature of, 74–75; order sets of, 107–108; reason for examination (RFE) for, 81–82, 107

Chief information officers (CIOs), 268; as committee chairpersons, 61; as committee members, 56, 57, 58; vendors as, 64. *See also* Chief medical information officers (CMIOs)

Chief medical information officers (CMIOs), 54–55, 57, 268; role in change control, 220, 222–223

Cholesterol-lowering drugs, 17

CIOs. *See* Chief information officers (CIOs)

"Circling back" training method, 148, 155, 165

Clarke, Arthur, 189

Clinical decision support (CDS), 245–265; add-ons for, 248, 249, 251; asynchronous, 247, 248, 258, 277; as cloud-computing, 250; as computer device feature, 201–202; clinician-designed, 249–250; definition of, 247; design and development of, 251–263; dynamic, 251, 271; effective, 252–253; key questions for, 256–263, 265; meaningful-use certification and, 252–253; as meaningful-use requirement, 174, 178, 252–253; need for, 246–247; oversight committees for, 252; poorly designed, 247, 248; predictive capability of, 250–251, 262–263; quality of, 249; root cause analysis in, 252, 253; rules for, 251–262; synchronous, 247, 249, 277; timing of, 261–262; well-designed, 247–248; types of, 248–251. *See also* Alerts

Clinical registries, 29

Clinical steering committees, 55, 56, 58–59

Clinical usability, of electronic health record systems. *See* Usability, of electronic health record systems

Clinics, electronic health record system implementation in, 210, 217, 230

Cloud computing, 250

CMIOs. *See* Chief medical information officers (CMIOs)

Codes, medical: exemption from computerized physician order entry (CPOE), 211; medication administration during, 67; un-tasked orders for, 51

Committee meetings, agendas of, 47–50

Committees: arguments/discussions within, 52–54; decision making by, 50; leadership of, 47–54; oversight, 60–62; prioritization by, 53–54; strategies for, 47–54; subcommittees of, 52–53; tasking behavior of, 50–52

Communication, 141–145; of agendas, 48; in change control, 221–222, 223–224; effective, 46; guidelines for, 142–145, 165; honesty in, 141; importance of, 140–141

Communication teams, 144–145

Computerized physician order entry (CPOE) systems: benefits from, 18, 19; big-bang and sequential approaches to implementation of, 206–212, 230; compliance with, 9–10, 18; definition of, 269; effect on physicians' workflow, 135–136; exemptions for, 210–212; functional phases of implementation, 206, 207–208; geographic phases of implementation, 206, 208–210; meaningful-use requirements regarding, 182–183, 184–185; natural language systems use in, 40; partial implementation, 210–212; percentage placed, calculation of, 182, 183, 184, 185; privileges for use of, 225, 226, 227, 257; serial and parallel orders in, 136, 275, 277; training in, 154; vision statements for, 9–10; in wireless infrastructures, 194–195

Computers, role in patient care, 6–7. *See also* Devices, used in electronic health record systems

Computers on wheels (COWs), 193, 211, 269

Confidentiality, of personal electronic devices, 191–192

Consultants: for leadership evaluation, 68–69; multiple, 245, 246; residents' contact with, 240, 241; role in patient care, 263; third-party, 33–34, 58, 63

Continuing medical education (CME) credits, for electronic health record system training, 161–162

Convenience order sets, 108–110, 113, 269

Conversion, to electronic health record systems. *See* Implementation, of electronic health record systems

Core measures, reportable, 186–187, 267, 278

COWs (computers on wheels), 193, 211, 269

CPOE. *See* Computerized physician order entry (CPOE) systems

CPSI, 37, 38

"Cry wolf problem," of alerts, 254, 269

C-suite, definition of, 269

Customization, standardization *versus*, 65–66

Data: collection of, 187; optimization of, 238–239; reliability and validity of, 237–238; sharing of, 29; viewing of, 135

Data display screens, 190–191, 196–197, 203

Deadlines, 46–47

Decision making: by committees, 50; documentation of, 241–243. *See also* Clinical decision support (CDS)

Decision support: definition of, 270; as electronic health record system function, 29. *See also* Clinical decision support (CDS)

Demographic data, meaningful-use requirements for, 173, 178

Department home folders, 90, 113–116, 117; definition of, 272; optimization of, 238; *versus* order sets, 116, 118; subfolders of, 114

of, 63–64; policy-and-procedure decisions, 66–68; risk *versus* workflow, 64–65, 69; standardization *versus* customization, 65–66; upfront work *versus* user work, 65. *See also* Leadership

Governance "tree," 55–56

Hardware: changes to, 62; maintenance of, outsourcing of, 63–64. *See also* Devices, used in electronic health record systems

Healthcare Information and Management Systems Society (HIMSS), website of, 280

Healthcare quality, *See* Quality, of healthcare

Health Information Technology for Economic and Clinical Health (HITECH) Act, 171–172. *See also* Meaningful-use requirements

Health information technology (HIT), use of, 4

Health IT Home website, 280

Healthland, 38

Heart failure, as reportable core measure, 186, 187, 272

Help lines, 218, 219–220, 230

Herodotus, 9

HIMSS Analytics, 5, 32, 41, 280

Historical documentation, 217–218

HMS, 38

Home folders. *See* Department home folders

Home medications default orders, 132

Honesty: in communication, 141; as leadership characteristic, 44–45, 46, 47

Hospitalists, order sets of, 113–114

Hospitals: health information exchange among, 174, 177; primary and secondary goals of, 169; purpose of, 3

IBM, 34

If-then orders, 86, 93, 272

Immunization registries, 29, 175, 180

Implementation, of electronic health record systems, 54, 205–230; bigbang and sequential approaches in, 206–212, 230, 267, 277; catalog cleanup during, 73; change control and, 220–224; change control and support for, 220–224, 230; common problems and solutions in, 64–68, 225–227; cost of, xi, 208; data viewing component of, 135; definition of, 272; documenting component of, 135, 136; duration of support for, 224–225, 229; examples of, 13, 14; failure of, 13, 14; functional phases of, 206, 207–208; geographic phases of, 206, 208–210, 272; go-live phase of, 272; governance of, 55–60, 69; help line support for, 218, 219–220, 230; importance of, 205–206; market for, 64; measurement of success of, 227–230; as medical project, 21; optimization following, 60–62; partial, 210–212, 275; placing orders component of, 135–136; preloading of clinical data prior to, 217–218; ratio and levels of support for, 219–220; rationale for, 3–8, 11–12, 24–25, 59; scheduling of, 213–217, 230; statements of purpose for, 7; support for, 218–227; support staff for, 213, 214, 219, 230; tips for success in, 15

Incentives, for electronic health record use, 4, 32, 218–219

Informal orders, 79–80

Informatics Review, xi

Information resources, for electronic health record systems, 279–281

Information technology (IT): definition of, 273; relationship to patient care, 263–264

Information technology projects: deadlines for, 46–47; implementation phase of, 54; leadership structures for, 54–68; medical perspective on, 3; optimization phase of, 54

Information technology steering committees, 56, 59

Information technology systems: clinical nature of, 54; specialized, 63. *See also* Electronic health record (EHR) systems

Inspector General, 6

Installation rate, of electronic health record systems, 39

Institute for Clinical Systems Improvement (ICSI), venous thromboembolism prophylaxis guidelines of, 235, 236

Institute of Medicine (IOM), *To Err Is Human: Building a Safer Health System*, 5

Intensive care unit (ICU) alerts, 254

Intensive care units (ICUs): as electronic health record system initial implementation site, 210; medication records in, 130; patient transfers in, 130

Interfaces, of electronic health record systems, 28; effect on user compliance, 236; limitations to and improvements of, 234–235; optimization of, 236

Internet, as information source: for electronic health record systems, 279–280; for medical information, 239–240

Intuitiveness, of electronic health record systems, 31

iPads, 191

iPhones, 201, 240

Jargon, avoidance of, 142–143

Joint Commission: clinical decision support rules and, 252; core measures of, 186–187, 267; definition of, 273; "ding" citations from, 252, 270; electronic health record system requirements of, 35; verbal orders confirmation requirement of, 211

Knuth, Donald, 231

Labor and delivery (L&D), electronic health record system implementation in, 210, 217

Laboratory data: meaningful-use requirements regarding, 174, 177; preloading of, 217

Laboratory systems, catalogs of, 72, 79

Laboratory tests: as catalog category, 72; orderable options lists of, 78

Laptop computers, 191, 199

Leadership: characteristics of effective, 43–46; of committees, 47–54; dysfunctional, 68, 69; effective, 43–69; efforts to improve, 68–69; for electronic health record system implementation, 55–60; evaluation of, 68–69; strategies for effective, 46–54; structures for effective, 54–68; "two-and-a-half" problem of, 44–45, 49–50

Length of stay (LOS): definition of, 273; as patient care quality marker, 170, 227–228

Litigation, fear of, 253. *See also* Malpractice

Long-term usage, of electronic health record systems. *See* Optimization

Lost orders, 208, 210

Macros: layered, 273; training in creation and use of, 146, 148, 155

Malpractice, 131, 208

McKesson, 38, 39

Meaningful-use requirements, 171–188; for advance directives, 175, 180–181; for allergy lists, 173, 176–177; for certification of electronic health record systems, 176; for clinical decision support rules, 252–253; for computerized physician order entry (CPOE) systems, 182–183, 184–185; for core objectives, 172, 173–174; data and report inaccuracy problems associated with, 184,

185–186; deadline for, 39; definition of, 171–172, 273; definition problems associated with, 184–186; for demographic data sets, 173, 178; for diagnoses lists, 173, 181; for discharge instructions, 173, 178; for drug interaction alerts, 182–183; for exchange of information among providers, 174, 177; funding for, 168; for laboratory data, 174, 175, 177, 181; for lists of patients by specific conditions, 174, 179; for medication lists, 173, 181–182; for medication reconciliation, 175, 182, 183–184, 226; menu objectives in, 172, 174–175; for patient-specific education, 175, 179; practical concerns regarding, 172, 176–186; for security, 177; for smoking history, 178; Stage 1, 172, 173, 176–185; Stage 2, 172; Stage 3, 172; for syndrome surveillance data, 175, 180; for vital signs and similar data, 173, 178; workflow effects of, 181–184

Medical Education in the United States and Canada (Flexner Report), 4

Medical errors, causes of, 5–6; inappropriately named orderables, 74; order sets, 99; root cause analysis, 252, 253, 276

Medical errors, experienced by Medicare patients, 6

Medical errors, prevention of, 5; with chart signing requirement, 65; with clinical decision support, 247; as electronic health record system function, 29

Medical executive steering committees, 55, 58–59, 110–111

Medical information, sources of, 239–240

Medical knowledge, specialization of, 245–246

Medical orders, as computerized physician order entry (CPOE) exemption, 211

Medical students, motivation of, 12

Medicare patients, medical errors experienced by, 6

Medication: administration routes for, 77–78; interaction alerts regarding. *See* Drug–drug interaction alerts

Medication administration records (MARs): during implementation of electronic health record systems, 208, 210, 217; paper-based orders *versus*, 208; preloading of, 217

Medication disclaimers, 131

Medication errors: administration route–related, 77–78; as errors of commission, 98; as errors of omission, 98, 106; prevention of, with dose range checking, 84

Medication history: entry into electronic health record systems, 128; unclean, 278

Medication lists: meaningful-use requirements for, 173, 181–182; paper-based, 208

Medication orders, electronic: for new drugs, 83; order sets of, 98; paper-based orders *versus*, 208; prechecked, 106; prohibition of prechecked, 98, 106; standard *versus* nonstandard, 66; up-front work *versus* user work issue in, 65

Medication process teams, 73–74

Medication reconciliation: "complete," 131; definition of, 273; during discharge process, 131–132; meaningful-use requirements for, 175, 182, 183–184, 226; "partial," 131–132; as workflow issue, 182, 183–184, 226

Medication records: in patient transfers, 129–130; as workflow issue, 129–130

Meditech, 38, 39

Meds rec. *See* Medication reconciliation

Meetings: agendas of, 47–50; time limits for, 48–49

Microsoft, 29

Reverse allergy checking alerts, 257–258

RHOs (remote hosted organizations), 63–64, 190, 276

Risk, workflow *versus*, 64–65, 66–68, 69, 98

Root cause analysis (RCA), 252, 253, 276

Rounds, workflow in, 241

Royal Canadian Mounted Police, 8–9

Scheduling, of implementation, 213–217, 230. *See also* Timing

Screens, for data display, 190–191, 196–197, 203

Sebelius, Kathleen, 24

Security: as meaningful-use requirement, 174, 177; in personal electronic device use, 191–192

Sequential approach, in electronic health record system implementation, 206–212, 230, 267, 277

Serial orders, 137, 277

Serology, nomenclature of orderables in, 76

Server maintenance, outsourcing of, 63–64

Shakespeare, William, 205

Siemens, 38

Signatures, electronic, 135

Site visits, for vendor evaluation, 36–37

"Smart rooms," 193

Smoking cessation advice, 187

Smoking history, as meaningful-use requirement, 173, 178

Social intelligence, 44

Software: changes to, 62; disparity with workflow, 122–123; maintenance of, outsourcing of, 234; for optimization, 238–239; updates to, 234. *See also* Add-ons

Specialists, responsibility for medication reconciliation, 131–132

Specialization, of medical knowledge, 245–246

Specialties, standard of care–based order sets of, 92–93, 111

Staff: attitudes toward electronic health record systems, 10, 12, 14, 39; dedication to patient care, 12–13; interface with electronic health record systems, 28–31; role in electronic health record system implementation, 7; vendor preferences of, 38–39. *See also* Nurses; Physicians

Standardization: customization *versus*, 65–66; order sets–based, 91–101, 116; protocol-based, 92

Standards, clinical, evidence-based, 234, 236

Standards of care, as basis for order sets, 92–93, 111

Standing orders, 80–81, 277

Stat orders, in emergency departments, 129

Stool cultures, order sets for, 107

Stress, 224–225

Stroke, as core measure, 186, 277

Subcommittees, 52–53

Super-users, of electronic health record systems, 156, 157–158, 218, 219, 230, 277

Support staff, for electronic health record system implementation, 213, 214, 219, 230

Surgery: electronic health record system implementation scheduling for, 217; exemption from computerized physician order entry (CPOE), 211

Surgical Care Improvement Program (SCIP), 186, 187, 276

Syndrome surveillance data, meaningful-use requirements regarding, 175, 180

Synonyms, clinical, of orderables, 76, 77

Tablets, 191–193, 211

Tasking, 50–52, 69

Team approach, in medicine, 263

Technology curve, 199–200

Templated documents, 241–242; use in wireless infrastructure, 194–196

Terminology. *See* Nomenclature rules

Text messages, 240, 241

Thompson, Fred, 167

"Three Ps," 225–226, 277

Thromboembolism, venous. *See* Venous thromboembolism

Timing: of change control, 222; of clinical decision support, 261–262; of communication, 143; of implementation, 214, 216; of training, 139–140, 148–150, 154–156, 159; of workflow, 123. *See also* Scheduling

To Err Is Human: Building a Safer Health System (Institute of Medicine), 5

Training, in electronic health record system use, 8, 31, 42, 200; "circling back" method of, 148, 155, 165; clinical nature of, 145–146, 165; competency assessment after, 155–156; cost of, 159–160; in documentation, 146, 148, 154–155; effect of implementation scheduling changes on, 215; guidelines for, 150–162; importance of, 139; inducements for, 161–162; insufficient, 145, 147–148; issues in, 162–165; needs analysis for, 159–161; of nursing staff, 153, 154; optimal, 147–148; of physicians, 154; physician-to-trainee ratio in, 151–153; policy issues in, 140; preparations for, 139–140; problems in, 145; required, 161; resources for, 150, 156; as retraining, 231–232; syllabus for, 150–153, 165; timing of, 139–140, 148–150, 154–156, 159; trainers, 156–158, 159, 162, 164; types of, 157–158; web-based, 157, 158, 278

Training domains, 159–161

Triage orders, 184–185, 278

"Two-and-a-half" problem, 44–45, 49–50

"Unfunded mandates," 65

United States Department of Health &
Human Services, 4, 24; Health IT Home website of, 280

United States Postal Service, 9

Up-front work, *versus* user work, 65

Usability, of electronic health record systems, 10, 24, 28, 29–31, 39, 42; of electronic devices, 190–193, 197, 198, 200–201, 202; factors affecting, 30; optimization in, 234, 237–239, 243–244

User work, *versus* up-front work, 65

Variance, in patient care, 65–66

Vendors, of electronic health record systems, 278; best practices–related services of, 236; certification of, 176; of computer devices, 198; consulting and optimization focus of, 63, 64; hospitals' dependence on, 190; implementation scheduling and, 213; in information technology governance market, 63, 64; of order sets, 96, 98–101; support for meaningful-use requirements by, 176; technical improvements offered by, 234–235; as trainers, 156–157, 158

Vendors, of electronic health record systems, evaluation of, 23–24; checklist approach to, 25; clinical perspective in, 28–31; criteria for, 34–36, 42; future clinical technologies consideration in, 40, 42; initial and long-term support issue in, 39–40; of large vendors, 27–28, 37–38, 39; of midsize vendors, 38; of niche system vendors, 25–27; site visits for, 36–37; third-party consultants and, 33–37; of top-ranked vendors, 37–38

Venous thromboembolism: prophylaxis guidelines for, 235, 236, 255; as reportable core measure, 186, 187, 278

Verbal input, to information technology systems, 40, 62, 63

About the Authors

Michael B. Fossel, MD, PhD, has been involved in medical IT for the past decade and has worked full time for Cerner Corporation (a major EHR vendor) and HPG Resources (a consulting firm), in both cases as a physician executive and an IT consultant for hospitals. His experience consulting—on both EHR implementation and optimization—at more than 100 hospital systems throughout North America is unparalleled for providing a breadth of experience and perspective on the field.

Dr. Fossel was a clinical professor of medicine and a practicing emergency department physician for 25 years. He completed his PhD and MD at Stanford Medical School, where he taught courses and was the recipient of a National Science Foundation Graduate Research Fellowship. Dr. Fossel was the chief editor of a medical journal and has authored several medical books, including *Cells, Aging, and Human Disease* (Oxford University Press 2004), and more than four dozen academic articles on medicine, aging, and ethics for the *Journal of the American Medical Association, In Vivo,* and other academic journals. He has lectured at the National Institutes of Health and at universities worldwide and has been a frequent guest with PBS, the BBC, and other global and national media.

Susan Dorfman, DHA, is an accomplished healthcare innovations and marketing executive, a published author, and an industry speaker with strong ties to the healthcare and life sciences fields. Dr. Dorfman completed her doctorate in health administration with a strong focus on Health 2.0. She is currently serving as the chief marketing and innovations officer at CMI/Compas, the largest healthcare-focused media-buying and planning company in the United States.